NUTRITION FOR ENLIGHTENED PARENTING

Nutrition
for Enlightened Parenting

Marie-Laure Valandro

Lindisfarne Books | 2014

2014
Lindisfarne Books
An imprint of SteinerBooks / Anthroposophic Press, Inc.
610 Main Street, Great Barrington, MA 01230
www.steinerbooks.org

NOTE: many of the translations cited have been revised.

Book and cover: William Jens Jensen
Cover images © by the author

LIBRARY OF CONGRESS CONTROL NUMBER 2014948837

ISBN: 978-1-58420-169-4 (paperback)
ISBN: 978-1-58420-170-0 (eBook)

Contents

Part 1:   Initiation through Foods   1

Part 2:   Mother Earth—Her Food, Her People   58

Part 3:   Conclusion: Future Lands   181

Bibliography   189

Dedicated to Paul and Fiorenza

The bread is not our food.
What us in bread does feed
is God's eternal Word,
is spirit and life indeed.[1]

"*Spirit is behind everything material. Thus, there is spirit behind all matter we take in through our nutrition;…by means of nourishing ourselves with this or that, we enter a relationship with something spiritual, a substrate behind the material.*"[2]

"*Someday we will learn to view earthly substances as processes come to rest, as the ancients did when they used the term 'end of God's paths.' Then we will see the specific qualities of a substance (its 'signature') as a free force, not necessarily attached to matter, whose place of origin is some distant point in the universe. The starry world radiates energies and qualities that fall on Earth and are condensed into substances here. These same energies and qualities also function here, on the level of living processes, as etheric, formative forces.*"[3]

"*Human beings simply cannot be thought of as combustion engines that are kept running by a certain amount of fuel, the energy output of which can be calculated in advance; rather, they are the scene of an interchange between cosmic and earthly forces.*"[4]

"*In earlier times, people had a healthy instinct for what was good for them. Long ago, when group-soul ties still united people, priests and leaders in the mysteries guided them in nutrition as in other matters. Now the time has come for guidance and instinct to be replaced by knowledge. However, striving for knowledge exposes seekers to error, on the one hand, and to dogmatism on*

1   Anonymous, from an ancient manuscript.

2   Steiner, quoted in Schmidt, *The Essentials of Nutrition*, p. 49.

3   Hauschka, *Nutrition: A Holistic Approach*, p. 182.

4   Ibid., p. 56.

the other. This explains why chaos reigns in knowledge—and in nutrition—today."[5]

"Eating and drinking are done every day on impulse or instinct. It actually takes a long time before those who are evolving spiritually include these things in their spiritual life.... Eating and drinking will be included only when we understand why we need to ingest physical substance rhythmically to serve the entire world's progress. Moreover, we must understand the relationship between physical substance and a spiritual life, as well as the ways in which our metabolism is not just physical but also spiritual because of its rhythms. 'In this way' we develop the habit of not just allowing eating to be a physical fact; we also form the habit of recognizing the role played, for example, by the spirit when a fruit ripens in the sunlight."[6]

"Humanity today does not need rules but knowledge and insight; not fixed traditions but the development of new capacities; not an escapist 'key to the Kingdom of Heaven' but the ability to carry the spiritual into the earthly realm."[7]

"Everything brings health, which causes people to make themselves a center of creativity and production."[8]

"Through its very nature, spiritual knowledge transforms itself into love."[9]

"Love is the result of wisdom reborn in the 'I.'"[10]

"With the same necessity with which any event of nature takes place—whether an earthquake, eruption, or any other natural

---

5   Ibid., p. 17.

6   Schmidt, *The Essentials of Nutrition*, p. 296.

7   Ibid., p. 299.

8   Steiner, quoted in Schmidt, *The Essentials of Nutrition*, p. 303.

9   Steiner, *An Outline of Esoteric Science*, p. 397.

10 Ibid.

event, great or small—two human beings meet in life according to the paths in life they have taken."[11]

"Our physical and etheric bodies have come to us from divine-spiritual worlds and divine-spiritual beings. Consequently, we should not view them with arrogance and condescension, but with holy reverence."[12]

"What do we really know? First, we know what we have learned from experience. This is all we know and nothing else!"[13]

"It is a delight to read how he [a person with sensitive feeling for the world of nature] sits at a table eating bread and vegetables while contemplating the ways of the airy element, the falling of fructifying rain, the roughness of ploughed fields, the Sun's capacity to ripen things. One rejoices in the apple's roundness, the glorious array of color in a fruit bowl, the pretty crockery, the clean white tablecloth. These pleasurable thoughts awaken one's deepest gratitude and love. A ceremonial mood envelops the scene, and the writer calls it a 'feast of embodiment,' Such a one would have us realize that being fed involves both spirit and body, that it is communion between Heaven and Earth celebrated by and in human beings."[14]

11 Steiner, *Karmic Relationships*, vol i., p. 39.

12 Steiner, *Esoteric Lessons, 1904–1909*, p. 404.

13 Steiner, *Esoteric Christianity*, p. 242.

14 Hauschka, *Nutrition*, p. 29.

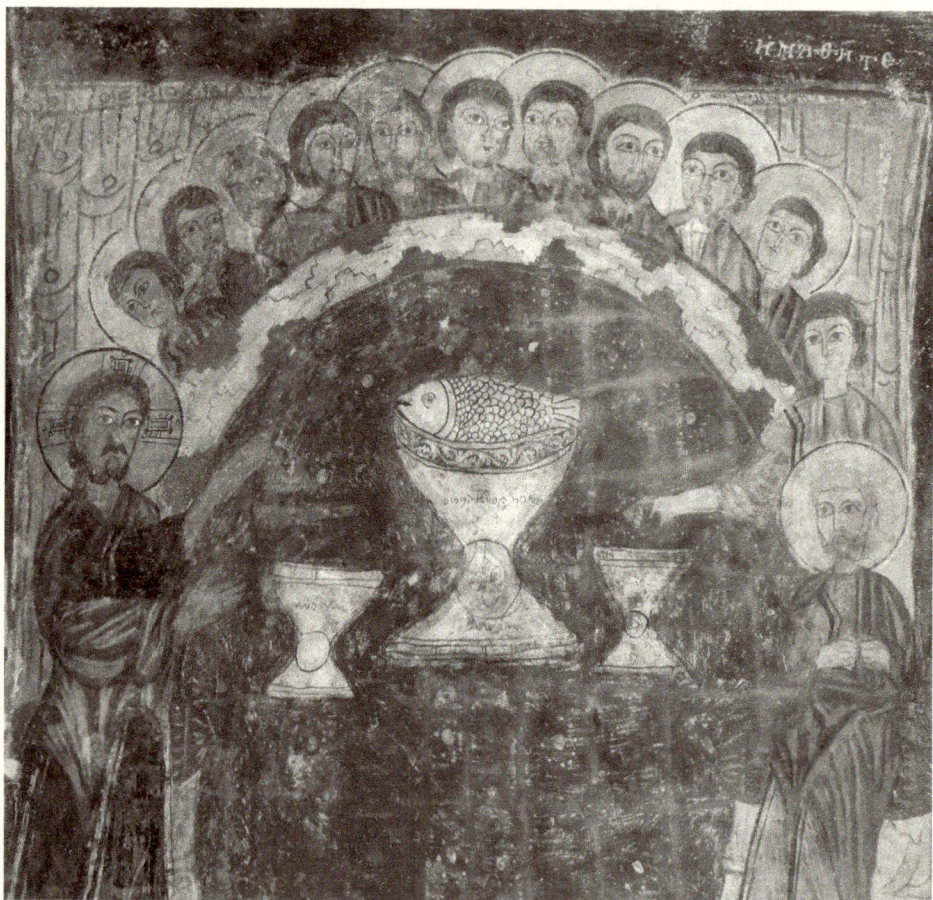

An image of Christ and the Disciples feeding the multitude
(Gulsehir Aciksaray, St. Jean Church, Cappadocia, Turkey, 13th century)

Part 1: Initiation through Foods

"I lost fifty pounds!" my friend said to me as I looked at this transformed woman whom I had met several years earlier. She and her husband are neighbors of mine for part of the year where I live in an idyllic hidden valley in the Canadian Rockies, the land of the far north surrounded by a circle of tall peaks reaching majestically toward the heavens, with the Columbia River close by, meandering through them. I come here to write and live as a hermit, but my neighbors are a welcome warmth to my solitary ways. I had not seen her for a few months, so I was taken by surprise.

To lose so much weight in a few months is very difficult, but she had to. The doctors told her that she was pre-diabetic and she needed to change, otherwise she would have many complications. She is in her mid-fifties. So she quit her job and started to seriously change her eating habits, to transform herself. She went through a regimented diet to avoid diabetes: nothing refined including sugar, no meat, eggs, milk or cheese, but wholesome foods such as grains, one tablespoon of olive oil per day, and legumes for her proteins. She became vegetarian, adopting a Hindu diet more or less, and the diet of most people in the Middle East, except that they eat lamb and other meat. She ate lots of chickpeas and lentils for protein, and she could eat pasta, bread, and cereal. One can look up this kind of diet in all sorts of books.

As we were chatting, she said, "Before I lost all this weight, I had a very hard time getting up in the morning. My body did not react. I was lethargic, and my extremities were bloated. Now I am up, I have much more energy, and I feel like myself again. And I can go for walks."

I was delighted. It was partly selfish, because I wanted her to return to downhill skiing so I would have a companion, and she is a barrel of laughs, besides being one of the finest psychologists I have ever encountered. She works in healthcare services in a large city, serving those who have been forgotten by society. Her caseload is in the hundreds: drug addicts, alcoholics, women abandoned by their mates, indigenous Indians lost in modern life, new refugees from Africa and elsewhere, Moslem women in a society strange to them. She pours her love and care out to the people who come to her. She listens to these human beings without judgment and honors their dignity. But the load was too great and her health had suffered, so she came to the mountains to refill her soul with strength, courage, and enthusiasm.

Her willpower in determining her future is remarkable. My friend, like many others in our Western society of plenty, has chosen a path to transform herself. It is an initiation into freeing ourselves of obsessions, of instinctual behavior, and one in which we regain control—control over food. This is all about freedom—freedom to determine what *we* want, not our bodily desires, instincts, and needs. It is a long path, but in the end we are the winners as we determine our own destiny; we become the ones in charge. Now, obviously, my friend was in charge of her life, and her energies were back.

> In the remote past, during their first incarnation on Earth, human beings were entirely under the sway of every emotion and desire; although they had an "I," they behaved as animals behave. The difference between a wild individual and a highly evolved idealist lies in the fact that the former has not yet worked through the "I" upon the astral body [emotion and desire body]. The next step in evolution is for human beings to work on their astral body. The result of such work is that certain fundamental properties of the astral body are brought under the individual's own control....
>
> The essential characteristic of the pupil's initiation is this: learning is regarded as a mere preparation; much more is done for initiation when the temperament itself is transformed. If a feeble

memory has been changed into a strong one, if violence has been changed into gentleness, a melancholic temperament into serenity, more has been accomplished than the acquisition of great learning. Herein lies a source of inner, esoteric powers, for this indicates that the "I" is working upon the ether body [life body], not only upon the astral body.[1]

Through this initiation, this great struggle, one can learn again "the power to read in the great Book of nature" through the foods we eat, what stands behind what we eat, and the spiritual within material substances. We need to regain an awareness of *what* it is we are eating and be able to say yes or no to it. We will benefit from regaining an appreciation of substances if we dive into them and try to understand their "work," and be thankful for the selflessness of the mineral, plant, and animal worlds. Then we can truly be caretakers of these worlds instead of irresponsible takers. That is the intention of writing such a book as this, to help follow this path through food.

In the West we live in a society of plenty—plenty of material wealth but internal emptiness—and it shows. I am reminded of a story about a lady from Paris who lives alone with no visits from children or friends in this very cosmopolitan, wealthy city. She was explaining her loneliness to her adopted friend, a single Moslem lady from a tiny village in the middle of nowhere in southern Tunisia adjacent to the Algerian border. I was invited to lunch at this very modest home at the edge of the Sahara Desert where the extended family lives in a few rooms. This lady from Paris now comes to this place for a few months every year. Here she has found friends, love, and care through her acquaintance with this remarkable woman. Her friend even wanted her to move permanently from the solitude and loneliness of the Western affluent city to this village. Here the people have few material things but plenty of heart, warmth, and love for others. We had a lovely heart-to-heart conversation when I was there.

---

1   Steiner, *Rosicrucian Wisdom: An Introduction*, pp. 19–20.

In the West, people have gained enormous amounts of weight, demonstrating the imbalance within their very own bodies. We could say we are undergoing an initiation, a massive initiation. Other initiation paths are not so obvious, such as psychological disorders, alcoholism, or drug consumption, but being overweight or underweight cannot be hidden. We must carry the burden around for everyone to see, which makes it excruciatingly painful for all concerned.

We take in food consciously when we eat to live or unconsciously when we live to eat. So, leaving aside the problem of over-consumption of foods, what is behind the foods we eat? Now come many questions: How does food affect us? What really happens when we digest our food? What really feeds us? What happens if we choose one diet over another? Meat or no meat? How about raising our children? What happens if we decide to feed our children a meat diet as opposed to a vegetarian one? What lies behind all of these choices?

I will draw from my knowledge of Spiritual Science, of Anthroposophy, as given to us by the seer and scientist-philosopher Rudolph Steiner and some of his brilliant students who followed his indications in medicine, agriculture, and the meditative life. I am deeply thankful for Dr. Hauschka's books on substances and nutrition, and I will quote from them extensively. He shows knowledge unmatched by contemporary nutrition experts. He loved the Earth, and it shows in his research and poetic writings. Gerhard Schmidt, a doctor and nutrition scientist, has also carried out extensive up-to-date research on nutrition. Karl König, another scientist, will be mentioned as well in regard to his genius in many fields of knowledge related to nutrition, agriculture, animals, plants, and earth science. Some of his insights will seem revolutionary, but that is what we need.

The old ways of looking at food are completely lost to our Western society. In other parts of the world where traditions are still alive, it is not so much of a problem, but they, too, will suffer as they lose their old ways. As one travels this Earth one can see this. It is, perhaps, the price we pay for the responsibility of freedom. We are no longer guided by rules handed down from generation to generation for our dietary needs. We eat whatever we please, whenever we please. In this freedom, we often choose wrongly because we sometimes place our desires ahead of what is good for us. The "looks good, tastes good" wins, and the body loses. That is a price of freedom.

But in this dietary revolution we are undergoing now—one that reflects our chaotic environment in all spheres of life—we are confronted with choices. More important, we have the opportunity to grow. We have the chance to truly become individuals who think and learn about our bodies, our souls, and our spirits. Food is a challenge, especially when we realize that most of planet Earth suffers from hunger, massive hunger. Fat versus starvation is the great imbalance on our Earth, and it is a reflection of things to come.

Initiation through food could lead us to think of those less fortunate, and perhaps we might start a fund by putting aside some of the money for foods we decide not to buy or eat. It could be sent to the truly needy of our world—extra fat saved for the hungry.

Raising a family and choosing the family's diet provide powerful tools for change and bringing health into the world. The domain of the home, of homemaking, cooking, caring once again, can become sacred, artistic activities that fulfill the soul and bring dignity to lost arts. These domestic realms have been ignored and forgotten by our materialistic society. The ordinary housewife is relegated to the end of the line. People might say, "Oh, you are a housewife, how nice," while really thinking, "Poor thing. What a life!"

I encountered this often after I decided to stay home and give up my profession. A cocktail party encounter with professional men and women often went like this: "What do you do?" a surgeon asked me, looking smart in a black dress. I answer with enthusiasm, looking equally good in my smart dress (on purpose, of course), "I am a housewife." The conversation stops, and then—if the person is not too haughty and full of his- or herself, with a Dr. beside the name—I go on to step two of the conversation. "But after I have done my housewife work, because I do not scrub the floors all day you know, I also work as a translator, I paint, write, teach skiing, garden, am a trained herbalist, take care of two children, and I just got back from a trip to southern France, where I filmed a documentary on an important writer living there." The surgeon does not feel so hot now, and maybe she is thinking, *Hey, she has a better life than I do. I do not know my kids, because I am never home. They are having all sorts of problems at school. I do not even know how to cook. I don't have the time. Perhaps I should work less. She is a housewife and she does not look that dumb. And she has a life while I only have a life at the hospital. And I am also worn out.* Then we might reach step three in the conversation, about cooking and canning, and she might just learn how to do some of these things. She might begin taking time out, and it might occur to her that she is sacrificing an enormous amount—her womanhood—by being a professional surgeon. Our society does not allow women the freedom to enjoy both children and work, but one must be sacrificed, and it is usually the children. Where is the middle ground?

Returning to our subject, what we will look at in this book is truly revolutionary, and it will require attention. It is not easy to understand, but with determination and good will, processes will become clear.

Can we bring up children in a way that will help them become free human beings so they realize their true destiny? How can we do this? Can we help or hinder by the way we choose to feed them? How we feed children is the other topic that will take on new meaning. How can we feed children in a way that fosters independent thinking? Or, looking at the question the other way around: in choosing a particular diet do we bring up human beings with a slave mentality? Will they be slaves to external circumstances such as drug addiction, drinking, sexual needs, foods, pain, sensual enjoyment, computers, and extreme sports? Or do we bring up strong individuals who can determine their own lives?

Can we help children by choosing foods wisely as we prepare our family meals? What are some other ways of feeding children? We can provide the best education for our children, but if they go home and eat a certain diet, perhaps even the best education will not be adequate. On the other hand, we can feed children the best diet with homegrown biodynamic food, whole milk, vegetarian or non-vegetarian with our own meats and eggs. But if we do it without food to feed the senses, then what happens?

Let us start from one beginning:

> The embryo will be affected if the expectant mother is not properly nourished; for its sake the mother must be cared for. Similarly, what later still surrounds and protects the child must also be cared for, as that in turn will benefit the child. This holds good on both physical and spiritual levels. Thus, as long as the child still slumbers as if within an etheric womb and is still rooted in the astral covering, it matters greatly what happens in the environment. The child is affected by every thought, every feeling, every sentiment motivating those nearby, even if not expressed. Here a person cannot maintain that one's thoughts and feelings do not matter as long as nothing is said.
>
> Even in the innermost recesses of their hearts, those around a child cannot permit themselves ignoble thoughts and feelings. Words affect only the external senses, whereas thoughts and feelings reach the protective sheaths of the ether [life] and astral [feeling] bodies and pass over to the child....
>
> Therefore, as long as these protective coverings envelop children, they must be cared for. Impure thoughts and passions harm them just as unsuitable substances harm the mother's body.[2]

I will try to include these topics throughout this food journey— an international one that will lead to realms beyond our senses.

---

2   Steiner, *Supersensible Knowledge*, p. 103.

However, before the story unfolds, these words must be taken seriously:

> Now you know we have to be clear in our minds that the spirit exists; but to be able to play a role on Earth the spirit has to act in physical matter. And if we work with the science of the spirit we really must know how the spirit is active in physical matter.[3]

We will dive into different substances and processes and learn how the spirit comes down into matter via these substances. Hopefully the substances will become more familiar, like friends. Carbohydrates will not be merely "carbs" but something more; proteins will become also something more than proteins, and the same with fats. And the air we breathe and the minerals, plants, and animals that feed us will be seen in a different light. Putting a pill in one's mouth will feel a bit different after reading this book.

I was a born vegetarian, meaning that I rejected meat when I was a child. I remember being stuck at the table chewing meat and being unable to swallow it. It was repulsive and made me sick, but my parents, thinking of meat as essential, made me eat it. I would find all sorts of stratagems to get rid of it, giving it to the dog or going outside to spit it out, rather than spending what seemed like hours chewing what became a thick mashed substance that my body could not swallow. It was truly a hellish experience. Mine was a body that needed the vegetarian diet. I instinctively knew that meat was poison for me, and it was.

When we moved to Africa it was easier, and I did not have to eat meat. I escaped eating it because there were so many other good things to eat that it was not served too often. My parents by then were very busy and did not make such a fuss. We had two fig trees in our little backyard in Rabat, Morocco, and later in Annaba, Algeria, there were kilos of oranges that I gathered in my skirt

---

3   Steiner, *From Mammoths to Mediums...*, p. 282.

and ate sitting in the dirt in front of our apartment complex. So I mostly survived on oranges, figs, yogurt, pasta, couscous, bread, and cheese, but did not like tomatoes, cucumbers, mushrooms, or onions. North Africa was a saving grace for someone like me; it was sunny so I ate sunny foods.

When we returned to France I was twelve and then I had to go on a regular diet. Now I ate eggs, yogurt, cheese, pasta, and bread, but because I was somehow deficient in my diet, I craved sweets. I ate pounds of chocolate and candy, enormous quantities that ruined my teeth. I also had appendicitis at age thirteen as a direct result of this diet. Then we moved to the United States where the diet was atrocious, and my sisters and I had enormous difficulties with the food. To us it seemed tasteless. We did not consider cereal with cold milk to be fit for human consumption. It tasted like cardboard to us. We wanted nice French bread and butter—real food. But the United States in the 1960s seemed to have forgotten what real food was. At home, however, we cooked French food and maintained a good diet. I learned how to cook because I enjoyed it, and I began to eat a bit more meat. By this time I was a teenager so I would occasionally eat the famous American hamburgers.

Through this very different upbringing—changing diets several times in the first twenty-one years of my life—I became interested in food from the very beginning. I was conceived in Burgundy but born in Tunisia, which I recently visited for the first time. I only spent one year there, six months in my mother's womb and six months out, but I think that it was enough for me to be exposed to sunlight, the wonderful aroma of spices, fresh bread making, and couscous, one of my favorite foods. In the souk/lively bazaar, which my mother walked through to get to work, I took in all of this, before birth and after. I feel much at home in such environments.

> We can say that the way the head of a pregnant woman is stimulated is strongly connected with her child's development.... What a

woman does with her head during pregnancy becomes the source of the activity taking place in her womb. She shapes and forms the child with what she imagines, feels, and wills.[4]

My grandmother on my father's side was Italian, and she was a great cook. I learned about pasta making from scratch by spending much time in her kitchen as I was growing up and watching her from my small stature, barely able to see the large tabletop upon which she would make the pasta—cutting it into long strands for noodles, amid a cloud of flour. To me, watching her move about her kitchen with its shiny copper pots was a sacred activity that touched me inwardly and guided my connection to food and cooking.

I remember sitting at her breakfast table, and then she would take us on a delightful adventure to the basement to get wonderful varieties of new jam. The basement was large and carefully lined with shelves of jars: cherry, strawberry, and plum, my favorite. She made everything. We spent hours in the spring and summer on her properties—our house was part of her large estate—and we walked on the little paths lined with strawberries and vegetables she had planted. We climbed all the trees and stuffed ourselves with cherries, plums, and other fruit. It is no wonder I did not eat meat. She cooked polenta with tomato sauce and rabbit, which I did not mind. She made *knokies*, a kind of delicious potato dumpling that I was never able to replicate. I grew up within this lifestyle until I was six.

On weekends we would travel quite a distance through winding roads into the Burgundy countryside to reach the farm of my grandfather on my mother's side, which was pure French, stemming from old Burgundian stock. There was no access, no road, so we had to make our way on barely passable dirt paths through rocky fields where red poppies and bluets grew in the summer. There it was bare essential eating. My grandfather had twelve children, my mother being the eldest. He farmed with horses, worked in the woods to cut

---

4   Steiner, *From Comets to Cocaine...*, p. 160.

firewood, had milking cows that some of his daughters milked, and a flock of sheep that his other daughters kept along with German shepherds and chickens. He grew his own peas, potatoes, and other vegetables that I helped him plant while sitting in the dirt when I was barely old enough to stand. To me it was wonderful, never mind that there was hardly any food to eat. They made potato soup and a milk soup with bread in it, ate Camembert, and a little chocolate for sweets. They had basically no meat and few vegetables. They walked to the small village down the little mountain through a forest path to buy enormous loaves of bread. I loved those walks, and they were the beginning of my love affair with walking. I could feel the little invisible beings everywhere on the moss-covered path deep in the forest. Those early experiences have led me to journey thousands of miles on foot around our planet Earth. My small legs became accustomed to walking, and now my older legs still carry me on paths of wonder.

This remarkable "starvation diet" by our standards sustained my grandfather who lived until 88, the same age my mother is now. The other side of the family, my father's, all died soon after reaching 63, including my father. In my own family I can see the results of various diets and how they affect offspring. I take after my mother's side, and my sisters take after our father's. I am basically vegetarian, but will eat meat when it is offered, red meat less often. My sisters on the contrary have a mostly meat diet and they struggle with weight gain and health issues. Furthermore, within my family, I have three sisters born and raised in Europe and Africa and one sister born in the United States. My American sister has a completely different diet than the rest of the family, and food is not important to her. I can see that heredity plays an enormous part in the diet we choose, going back many generations. In the same family we will find vegetarians along with meat eaters. How do we address the needs of these very different individuals?

During a Buddhist meditation retreat I befriended a lady who had two sons. She was a strict vegetarian and brought up her boys on a vegetarian diet. One of the sons did very well; the other was sickly. She took him to a doctor who promptly told her to feed this boy a steak once a week. Unlike his brother, he needed meat in his diet. She quickly overcame her dogmatic vegetarian outlook and cooked meat for this little boy who soon grew as strong as his brother. I learned a lot from her. As a vegetarian myself at birth, I saw the other side of the story: a person was denied meat when his body needed it. Therefore, it is essential that mothers stay vigilant about their children's needs, whatever they may be. Children come to us from the spiritual world and will have different destinies which call for different diets. For example, one son is meant to be a business-man, and another son is meant to be a poet or musician. Who eats what? Your husband is of Chinese descent and you are Spanish. You are African American and your spouse is Irish. You are a bit heavy; she is super thin. You are Jewish; she is Japanese. He is Egyptian; you are German. This is our new world. Now, what about children?

My being a vegetarian from birth was, of course, not something I thought about. It was simply a fact. I could not stomach meat; it made me throw up and had nothing to do with my being aware of killing animals to eat them. I was too young to be concerned with such things. That came later. But as I grew older, it dawned on me that I am a vegetarian by birth because of my destiny, my past—past lives, past karma. Here some explanations are necessary to help us understand some of the problems we face when rearing children.

My body needed no meat; I was healthy without it. According to Rudolf Steiner, if we want to pursue spiritual and philosophical work we do better with a vegetarian diet. It keeps our bodies lighter and hardly burdens our digestive systems by loading them up with meats, which are heavy and leave residues in our bodies. We can then spend more time doing intellectual work. The meditative and idea realm is easier because the body is not encumbered with slug-gish digestion. In school it soon became apparent that I loved philos-ophy, comparative religious studies, literature, chemistry, languages, and so forth. And I did well in these realms. In my forties, I took up Spiritual Science full time along with my other duties as teacher, mother, wife, and artist. I still kept to the vegetarian diet throughout my pregnancies but included meat in the family diet because my husband was not a vegetarian.

I found that I could study with ease and was bewildered when others could not. I attribute this to my vegetarian diet, which did give me more energy for such studies as well as many other things. From my birth on, I knew my destiny. Or we can say from before birth when I specifically chose a body that would not like meat. Now I benefit from such a choice, by still being able to do enormous amount of work to the degree others cannot imagine. My friend's weight loss typifies the power of the vegetarian diet.

I am able to study, read, meditate, and keep a clear head thanks to a lacto-vegetarian diet with only occasional meat eating when I am traveling and no alcohol at all. I am a choleric by nature, sanguine sometimes, so not eating meat helps me in managing my hot temper. Having a fiery temper is not easy, believe me!

What happens when people exclude meat from their diets? The answer involves one of the revolutionary insights brought to our attention by Dr. Steiner. Counterintuitively, it is not easier on the body to be a vegetarian. It requires more forces to digest vegetarian foods such as legumes, whole wheat, and other unrefined foods than to digest meat, white flour, and white rice. We must have the forces within to digest unrefined, raw matter in the form of wheat, brown rice, quantities of vegetables, nuts, lentils, or chickpeas. Some people do not have the forces within their digestive system to do so and they fall ill. They need the meats, which are easier to digest than other basic foods.

The cow digests the grass, and we eat the meat which has already gone through the process of digesting the grass. When we eat greens we need to digest them, but it is easier on the digestive system to eat meat, because the digestive system does not work as hard. That is one characteristic. The other is that while our stomach works harder to digest a vegetarian diet, it grows stronger and we become more energetic as a result. The more our digestive system works, the stronger it gets; the more we feed it meat and refined foods, the lazier it gets. Therefore, we see sluggishness in people who consume enormous amount of meat and are overweight. It is this simple.

It is similar to exercising our muscles so they will grow stronger; if we don't they atrophy. So it is with the forces that are required to digest food: the stronger one's digestive system works, the more power it accumulates; therefore, there is more energy available from the breaking up of the food substances. The less work the digestive system takes on, the more lethargic we become.

Another revolutionary aspect of digestion which Rudolf Steiner spoke about in his many lectures has to do with what happens in the digestive system when we digest the food. We know the digestive system works harder, but what is really behind this fact? Steiner explained it in the following terms. I will quote several passages, so we can understand what happens from different angles.

> What happens then in the human being? In every moment something is happening in the human being which occurs nowhere else in our earthly surroundings. Human beings take in the foodstuff from the surrounding world. They take this food from the kingdom of the living and only to a small extent from what is dead. However, as it passes through the digestive system, it is completely destroyed. We take in living substance and completely destroy it, in order to infuse it with our own life. And not until the foodstuff passes into the lymph ducts is the dead made living again in our inner being.
>
> One can see, if one grasps the nature of the human being totally, that in the soul-and-spirit permeated organic process, matter is completely destroyed and then created anew. In the human organism we have a continual process of destruction of matter, so that matter can be newly created. Matter is continually changed into nothingness and newly created in us.

The door to this knowledge was firmly sealed in the nineteenth century, when people arrived at the law of the conservation of matter and of energy, and believed that matter is also conserved in the human organism. The establishment of the law of the conservation of matter is clear proof that the human being is no longer inwardly understood.[5]

Here we come to the crux, the heart of the matter, about our digestion. Again it is not easy to understand, but we must make the effort to grasp what is at stakes here. First, the digestive system works harder with a vegetarian diet, thereby releasing more energy, becoming stronger in the process. Second, the food we take in is destroyed, transformed to zero, to nothing. Then we recreate it. It follows the creation process: chaos must exist before creation is possible.

We must begin to understand what it is we do to our bodies when we choose what to eat. We owe it to our children not to be ignorant in this realm, as decisions that we make regarding our diet will have consequences for generations to come. If we choose to drink immoderate amounts of alcohol, the following generations will become weaker. That is a fact. Not just one generation is affected, but several. We would be responsible for breeding stupid offspring to put it bluntly—stupid, weak, unhealthy offspring. We can survive on the gene pool for a maximum of three generations. After that, the weaknesses take over, and the body is no longer able to be strong enough to endure an unhealthy diet and lifestyle and survive. In my case, thanks to my great-grandparents, grandparents, and parents who led relatively good lives, I am still healthy. But if these same great-grandparents were alcoholics, or had bad diets, then down the line, I would suffer from their bad diets and lifestyles. I would have a body prone to diseases or be mentally deficient. That is only one aspect of food and health. We

---

5   Steiner, *Becoming the Archangel Michael's Companions*, pp. 148–149.

will discuss this and much more, including choosing a vegetarian versus a meat diet.

But now, as you know, people not only eat plants; they eat animals, too—the animal's flesh, fat, and so on. Certainly it is never for Anthroposophy to assume a fanatical or sectarian attitude. Its task is only to tell how things are. One simply cannot say that people should eat only plants or that they should also eat animals, and so on. One can only say that some people with the forces they have from heredity are simply not strong enough to perform all the work within their bodies needed to destroy plant fats so completely that forces will then develop in their bodies for producing their own fat. You see, people who eat only plant fats—well, they have renounced the idea of becoming imposing and portly, or they must have awfully good digestive systems that are healthy enough for them to break down the plant fats and in this way get forces to build their own fat easily. Most people are really unable to produce their own fat if they have only plant fats to destroy. When we eat animal fat in meat, that is not entirely broken down. Plant fats do not go beyond the intestines, but are broken down within the intestines. However, the fat in meat does go beyond and passes right into the human being....

Therefore, we must distinguish between two kinds of bodies. First there are bodies that do not like fat; they don't enjoy eating bacon; they just don't like to eat fatty foods. Those are bodies that destroy plant fats relatively easily and want to form their own fat. They say: Whatever fat I carry around, I want to make it myself; I want my very own fat. However, if people heap their table with fatty foods, then they are not saying: I want to make my own fat. Rather, they are saying: The world must give me my bacon. Animal fat passes into the body, making the work of nutrition easier....

However, it is useless to be fanatical about such matters. There are those who simply cannot live without meat. People must carefully consider whether they actually can get along without it. If they decide they can do without it and change from a meat to a vegetarian diet, they will feel stronger than they were before. This is sometimes difficult, obviously; some people cannot bear the thought of living without meat. If, however, they become vegetarians, they feel stronger because they are no longer obliged to deposit alien fat in their bodies; they make their own fat, and this makes them feel stronger.

I know this from my own experience. I could not otherwise have endured the strenuous exertion of these last 24 years! I never could have traveled entire nights, for instance, and then give a lecture the next morning. It is a fact that those who are vegetarians carry out a certain activity within themselves that non-vegetarians are spared, since it is done first by the animal....

Whether we are able to become vegetarians or not is an individual matter.[6]

Growing up I remember all of us sitting at the family table eating, enjoying, arguing, talking, joking, and exchanging food from one plate to the other. I would give the fat to my father or sister who liked it. It was an easygoing exchange and no one made a fuss. I hated the fatty substances, and still do, but my sister relished them. I wondered how she could bear to eat them, but I learned to be tolerant at the table.

It should now become clearer that meat versus non-meat is more complicated than it seems. Now we expand upon what we mentioned before about the breaking down of foods to nothing, where none of the original substances remain. Let us look closer at this process of digestion, and as we enter into these realms more and more, we consider mysteries whose implications are far-reaching. These are long passages and they take a while to digest; one must read slowly and make pictures within one's mind. It takes effort, but the effort is worthwhile.

As foods pass through the digestive system they are progressively broken down and dissolved. They are first mechanically ground and moistened with saliva in the mouth through the chewing action. Then chemical activity sets in as glands of the mouth and throat are stimulated to secrete ptyalin and other substances.

---

6   Steiner, *From Sunspots to Strawberries*, pp. 94–96.

The pepsin secretions of the stomach are chiefly responsible for breaking proteins down into the form of peptones. Pancreatic secretions further reduce these to peptides in the small intestine and there continue the work of dissolution already begun by saliva in the mouth on fats and carbohydrates. Other intestinal secretions finally break up every ingested substance into the smallest, finest building material imaginable: proteins into amino acids, by way of peptones and peptides; carbohydrates into sugars; and fats into glycerine and fatty acids. The thoroughly dissolved chyme now passes by way of resorptive villi right through the intestinal wall and into the true digestive zone....

The breakdown of foods, which continues until they reach the intestinal wall, is essentially identical with that occurring in laboratory reduction of protein, carbohydrates, and fats when these are treated with retorts with appropriate reagents....

But what about further development on the other side of the intestinal wall?...

The etherealization of the chyme as it passes the intestinal wall and enters upon the first, completely non-material phase is perfectly analogous. The nutrient substances fade away, as it were, into the inner metabolic organism. And just as the cosmos brings forth a visible, substantial plant when it acts on the material anchorhold of the seed, likewise we create our own human substance (complete human protein) from equally non-material phases of nutrient substances through the agency of our digestive organs....

What actually happens when we digest our food? The foods fade, as it were, from the intestinal tract into the microcosmic space of the human being. Just as the Sun causes plants to spring up, blossom, pour out their fragrance, and decay, likewise we apply the strength of our personality to breaking down and gradually translating our nutrients into the non-material field of force that occupies the human microcosm. And exactly as the Sun, representing the cosmos, brings forth the new plant and its substances, likewise the "I" in control of the human microorganism and its forces creates its own body-building protein. Complete human protein is precipitated from human microcosmic substance by our human complex of forces, much as a sunny summer afternoon clouds over and a thunderstorm releases showers of rain from the lowering skies....

Digestion is thus the spiritualization of matter and stimulation of the personality forces to create new human substance. But it follows from this that digestion is a capacity of personality. It is therefore always an individual process, as individual as the bodily substances which it precipitates. No two human beings ever possess identical blood, for example. Everyone knows that two individuals fed exactly alike develop quite differently. One is easily satiated, the other always hungry; one is healthy, the other sick; one is fat, the other thin; one is smart, the other simple. This is reason enough to avoid dogmatism in nutritional matters![7]

Now we understand that the food we take in is totally destroyed as it becomes chyme. A further explanation of what happens involves an understanding of the breathing process that we are familiar with. We take in air, retain the oxygen, and breathe out carbon dioxide, which we cannot use but the plants can. We then eat the different foodstuff and obtain the carbohydrates (carbon-hydrogen-oxygen), the proteins, the fats, and the minerals. Rudolf Steiner explains this process involving carbon, something mainstream medicine does not even mention.

Let us suppose that we take into ourselves something of a mineral nature. Every such mineral substance must be so far worked on within the human being that the following results are brought about.... If you eat a grain of common salt, this must be absorbed by your individual warmth, not by the warmth which you have in common with the outside world. Your own individual warmth must take pleasure in absorbing it. Everything mineral must be transformed into warmth ether. And the moment people have something in their organism that prevents some mineral from being changed into warmth ether, at that moment they are ill....

Human beings take in plant substances; they, too, belong to the plant kingdom inasmuch as they develop the plant element in themselves. Mineral nature continually has the tendency to become

---

7   Hauschka, *Nutrition,* pp. 8–17.

warmth ether in humans. The plant element continually has the tendency to become airy, to become gaseous in humans. So that they have the plant element within themselves as a realm of air.... If it does not assume the form of air, if their organization is such that it hinders them from letting what is of a plant nature within them to pass over into the form of air, they become ill.... Everything of animal nature that humans take in or develops within themselves must...assume a fluid, watery form.... If human beings are not in a position to liquefy their own or foreign animal substance so as to recreate it again in a solid state, they become ill....

Everything mineral must eventually become warmth ether in the human being. Everything vegetable must undergo a transitional airy stage in humans. Everything animal must pass through an intermediate water stage in humans. Only what is human may always retain the solid earthly form within it. This is one of the secrets of the human organization....

If we follow the metabolism all the way through to the breathing process, we find that people release carbon dioxide, an element to be found everywhere in the human organism. This is sought out by oxygen and changed into carbon dioxide, which is then exhaled. Carbon dioxide is a compound of carbon and oxygen. The oxygen drawn in through breathing seeks out the carbon and absorbs it; carbon dioxide, the compound formed of oxygen and carbon, is then exhaled. But before it is exhaled, carbon becomes the benefactor, so to speak, of the human organism. Combining with oxygen, and therefore as it were combining what the blood circulation brings about with what the breathing then makes of the blood circulation, carbon becomes the benefactor of the human organization; for, before it leaves the human organization, it lets ether stream out everywhere in the organism. Physiologists merely state that carbon is exhaled with the carbon dioxide....People exhale carbon dioxide; but, due to the process of exhalation, ether is left behind everywhere in the organism; it is left by the carbon when it is claimed by the oxygen. This ether penetrates into a human's etheric body, and it is this ether, continually produced by the carbon, which makes the human organization capable of opening itself to spiritual influences, of absorbing astral and etheric impulses from the cosmos. The ether left behind by carbon attracts the cosmic impulses which in turn impose form principles on a human. They prepare the nervous system, for example, so that it can be a bearer of thoughts. The ether must continually be present in our senses, in our eyes, for example, so that they may be able to see, to receive the outer light ether. Thus we are indebted to carbon for the supply of ether within us that enables us to come into contact with the outside world....

What I really wished to show was that we must work on the mineral until it becomes warmth ether in order that it may absorb the spiritual; then, after the mineral has absorbed the spiritual, the human being can be built up by it.[8]

I can't help but think about carbon-diamond. If we know that carbon is the same substance as the diamond, then we can see how it is important in this process. It acts like the diamond in a way, in a subtle field of force—the forming force of the carbon, the end on Earth being the diamond. In a lighter more ethereal world our blood holds a diamond potential, taking in the forces from the cosmos right into our blood. It is an imagination that reminds me of the importance of this powerful substance: carbon.

Carbon is the "form-giving element" throughout nature. Carbon has a tremendous formative capacity for organizing and structuring matter in the physical world. It results in several millions of compounds. So we cannot be surprised that it has such an important function in the breathing process. Its formative function in the warmth ether is what helps us nourish ourselves.

It is utter nonsense to imagine that some mineral from the outside world would simply transfer itself into the human body and make up some part of the skeletal system, the teeth, etc. Before anything can be part of the human form it must have gone through the completely volatile warmth ether stage and then have been transformed again into a part of the living form of the human organism.

---

8   Steiner, *Harmony of the Creative Word*, pp. 165–195.

But something quite different is also connected with this: solid substance loses its solid form when it is changed in the mouth into fluid and is then transformed into the condition of warmth ether. It also gradually loses weight as it passes over into the fluid form and becomes more and more estranged from the earthly; but only when it has ascended to the warmth etheric form is it fully prepared to absorb into itself the spiritual which comes from above, which comes from cosmic breadths....

There is the mineral substance; this mineral substance enters into the human being. Within humans, passing through the fluid state, and so on, it is transformed into warmth ether. Now it is warmth ether. This warmth ether has a strong disposition to absorb into itself what radiates inward, streams inward, as forces from world spaces, from the breadths of the cosmos. Thus it takes into itself the forces of the universe. And these forces of the universe now become the spiritual forces which here imbue warmth-etherized earthly matter with spirit. And only then, with the help of this warmth-etherized earthly substance, does there enter into the body what the body needs to take shape and form.

So you see if, in the old sense, we designate heat or warmth as fire we can say: what humans absorb in the way of mineral substance is taken up to the level where it becomes of the nature of fire in them. And what is of the nature of fire has the disposition to take up into itself the influence of the higher hierarchies; and then this fire streams back again into all human's internal regions, and resolidifies to provide the material basis for the individual organs. Nothing that human beings take into themselves remains as it is; nothing remains earthly. Everything, and specifically everything that comes from the mineral kingdom, is so far transformed that it can take into itself the spiritual and cosmic; it then resolidifies into the earthly condition with the help of this.[9]

Carbon is the element which constantly goes through our body, helping in this process of bringing down the ether forces that come from the cosmos through its "magic" forming capacity. It is then

---

9   Ibid., pp. 184–185.

exhaled into the atmosphere, through our breathing, after having done its selfless work. It is truly a diamond. It is the heaviest substance in the air.

Carbon is present in carbohydrates (hydrogen, oxygen, carbon), in proteins (hydrogen, oxygen, carbon, nitrogen), and in fats. It is in tar's chemistry; it is everywhere. It is the earth substance in several million compounds. It is under the sign of Scorpio, the eagle forces in the cosmos, and is found in the forces of St. John's Gospel and "the word became flesh." Now Rudolf Steiner, through Anthroposophy, takes us on a further journey: "and the flesh is to become word." Carbon, as a selfless substance, was a plant and became dark, blackened coal, but it will become diamond once more and will still be a helper to humankind. Perhaps wearing a small diamond has its useful place in meditation. It has gone through a very long journey, and so is humanity's journey.

> This fact that we do not build ourselves up out of the earth and its matter but that we build ourselves up out of something that is beyond the earth. If it is the case that the whole body is renewed in seven years, the heart will also be renewed. So you no longer have the heart inside you now that you had eight years ago. It has been renewed, renewed not from the material substance of the earth but renewed out of the element that surrounds the Earth in the light. Your heart is compressed light! You really and truly have a heart that is condensed sunlight. And the food you have eaten has only given the stimulus for you to compress the sunlight so far. You build up all your organs from the light-filled surroundings, and the fact that we eat, that we take in food, only means that a stimulus is given.[10]

To understand this "condensed light" beyond physical substances, Steiner gives us this amazing passage from *Manifestations of Karma*.

> Spiritual research discovers a condition of dissolution in which all materials are reduced to a common basis, but what then appears

---

10 Steiner, *From Mammoths to Mediums*, p. 205.

there is no longer matter, but something which lies beyond all the specialized forms of matter around us. Every single substance, be it gold, silver, or any other substance, is there seen to be a condensation of this fundamental substance, which is really no longer matter. There is a fundamental essence of our material earthly existence, from which all mater comes into being only by a condensing process. The question: What is this fundamental substance of our earthly existence? is answered by Spiritual Science: Every substance on the Earth is condensed light. There is nothing in material existence in any form whatever which is anything but condensed light.... Wherever you reach out and touch a substance, there you have condensed, compressed light. All matter is, in its essence, light....

We have seen that light is the foundation of all material existence. If we look at the material human body, that also, inasmuch as it consists of matter, is nothing but a substance woven out of light. Inasmuch as human beings are material beings, they are composed of light....

Of what does the soul consists? If we applied the methods of spiritual scientific research to the actual basic essence of the soul we would find that everything that manifests on Earth as a phenomenon of soul is a modification, is one of the infinite variety of transformations possible, of that which we call love.... Every single stirring of the soul, wherever it occurs, is love modified in some way or other...we find that our outer corporeality is woven from light and that our inner soul is spiritually woven from love.[11]

So, we are woven out of light and love, wisdom and love. We have not strayed far away from carbon. Carbon is coal, fire, and the diamond is light, condensed light. It is present within us throughout our life, and it is necessary that we try to understand it. And now we have jumped into the mystery of nutrition, a complex journey.

I was a language teacher for many years, teaching French, Spanish, or English as a second language (ESL) in various countries, but

---

11   Steiner, *Manifestations of Karma*, p. 188.

especially in the United States. I made it my task to teach my students, usually ages thirteen to eighteen, to taste food from different countries, to actually taste another culture experientially. I taught in many small towns and rural farm areas, and these children sometimes resisted my attempt to introduce new foods into their diet. They all tried, however, when we turned the classroom into a kitchen or used the school's kitchen. It was an exercise in making them more pliable, not so set in their ways due to sclerotic home environments.

I remember taking a bus-load of forty-five children from rural northern Vermont where I taught to Quebec City with two other chaperones. I rented an entire youth hostel there, putting boys upstairs and girls downstairs, and made several reservations in classy restaurants. The children from poor farms and working areas had lunch or dinner in a candlelit atmosphere. They could sit with whomever they wanted and enjoy a meal of various delicacies they had never tasted before. They had the most wonderful time and never misbehaved, using lovely table manners. I still rejoice at the sight of these children learning about the Québecquois. They wandered around the city in groups of three or four and loved the experience of being somewhere else.

I wanted to encourage a few to become future travelers, and I hope I was successful. The cost was not exorbitant, and we raised the funds through cooking Spanish meals for the whole community. We served more than 150 people and ran out of food because it was so well received. I was twenty-four years old at the time. I subsequently took other bus-loads of high-school students from Connecticut and southern Vermont to enjoy their Quebec neighbors, always with the same success.

I had chosen this profession because it would allow me to make money right after college, as I was quite poor and had no one to fall back on except myself. I was going to graduate school in Middlebury, Vermont, where I found philosophers, poets, interesting friends, drama, and acting, and wonderful scholars as my professors. I had the summers off too, four glorious summers of books, lakes, quarries, mountains, and French Quebec just up the road.

As a teacher, I completely enjoyed the children as well as their parents and people in the community who were always welcoming. I taught in the Boston school system, which never liked my unconventional teaching methods. I was forever asking to use the auditorium for plays, or to go to the museum on the subway. The administration preferred that the kids sit in their classrooms, but I was not a sit-down kind of teacher. Naturally, when it came to renewing my contract they declined to do so. They hired someone who would sit behind the desk and not ask to constantly rock the boat. In my class the students were noisy, but enthusiastic. I taught in Boston, northern Vermont, southern Vermont, rural Connecticut, New Hampshire, Paris, Tehran, and Wisconsin. With all these children I always introduced cooking food as a means to teach new cultures and help them go beyond themselves. I tried to make them live into what it means to be a French man or woman, or a Spaniard, Mexican, or Columbian, to get them to go outside their skin and bring some movement into their soul lives. I must say after teaching all day I usually required perfect silence for a couple of hours before going on with my evening. These young people required an enormous amount of energy and nothing less than my total attention.

I remember telling the kids, during a cooking class, "Okay, pretend that you have had four cups of coffee. Act a bit nervous, fidgety, and speak French. Whatever comes out of your mouth does not matter; just use French words, verbs, or English words using a French accent." That was how we began. We broke the self-consciousness barrier immediately. Some actually seemed to look French! I also did not insist on correct verb endings, as they are too complicated for beginners. I would say, "Forget past, future, and present. Just speak." And little by little, as fear was abolished, the correct grammar would emerge. One cannot learn when one fears making a mistake. "Make a mistake and try again" was my art of teaching.

Actually, it's my art of living. No one is perfect, but one hopes to do better the next time. The point is to give it your best.

Where I am presently living, I find myself surrounded by former teachers, men and women who spent thirty to forty years in the classroom. They have come here because they love the outdoor lifestyle, with plenty of snow for skiing and mountains for hiking. Other "power" professions are not as lucky; they care for the sick, travel a lot, eat out, and lead a very out-of-rhythm life, which they pay for in their old age. Many like to merely sit and be entertained. But one finds that monetary success in the world is minimal compared to the success of regular teachers, loggers, mill workers, farmers, artists, and others who have to make do with much less money but make up for it with resourcefulness. The more artificial one's life is, the more disconnected from nature; the more intellectual, the more passive one becomes; and the more we are burdened by diet, weight, and illness problems, the more we must look to our lifestyles for the reasons.

It is actually true that in recent times people who really do not know what they want have become more and more numerous. It is indeed easy in our modern age for people not to know what they want because, for the last three or four centuries, the majority of them have become unaccustomed to occupying themselves with anything spiritual. They go to their offices and busy themselves with something they actually dislike but that brings in money. They sit through their office hours, are even quite industrious, but they have no real interests except going to the theater or reading the newspapers. Gradually, things have been reduced to this. Even reading books, for example, has become a rarity today.

That this has all come about is due to the fact that people don't know what they want. They must be told what they want. Reading the newspapers or going to the theater stimulates the senses and the intellect but not the blood. When one must sit down and read some difficult book, the blood is stimulated. As soon as an effort has to be made to understand something, the blood is stimulated, but people do not want that anymore. They quite dislike having to exert themselves to understand something. That is quite repugnant to people. They do not want to understand anything! This unwillingness to understand causes their blood to thicken. Such thick blood circulates more slowly. As a result, a remedy is constantly required to bring this increasingly thick blood into motion. It is brought into motion when they stick a cigarette into their mouth. The blood doesn't become thinner, but the blood circulation becomes ever more difficult. This can cause people to become afflicted with various signs of old age at a time in life when this doesn't have to occur.[12]

Reading this book will certainly require one to think, and it is meant to, to get the blood moving and perhaps make some changes in one's life, transform it. If one reader transforms his or her life, then my effort will have been worth it. This is called using one's *will*, and there is nothing more difficult—that is, when everything stands in the way of it (see *The Gentle Will* by Georg Kühlewind). "During our earthly existence we behold that which it pleases the Spiritual Beings to reveal to us."[13]

I have chosen to live in this area, the far north, and often wonder why I made this choice when I could have gone anywhere in the world. But I simply feel better here than elsewhere. I often hike up to 9,000 feet or more in the fall; in the winter I spend part of the day in the higher elevation, around 8000 feet, enjoying the snow and the high peaks. Recently I came across a very telling passage in one of Rudolf Steiner's lectures that made me think hard about this choice.

In recent years learned scientists have become more reasonable, and those with some sense have realized that it was not so long ago that everything here was covered with glaciers; in fact, all of Europe was still iced over when people in Asia were as clever as I have described, when the Babylonian and Assyrian cultures

12 Steiner, *From Comets to Cocaine...*, p. 223.
13 Steiner, *Karmic Relationships*, vol. 2, p. 223.

flourished. We need go back only a few thousand years—four or five thousand—to find that in Europe everything was still iced over. Only gradually, as the ice diminished, did human beings migrate here.

Well, these people did not have it as easy as people today. It was much harder on them, since they came from warmer regions where they were not constantly subjected to the cold and where they fared better. Nevertheless, these people did move into regions that only recently had been covered with ice. Through this they were prevented from experiencing the sensual pleasure of wisdom that would gradually have been theirs in Asia. Because an influence was exerted in Europe from the universe, causing it to be covered with ice when the Asian culture enjoyed a warm climate, a better, more energetic culture developed in Europe than could have evolved in Asia. You see, entire civilizations depend on influences from the cosmos....

In Asia there existed tremendously clever people who possessed strong soul natures. Gradually, however, they wanted to experience the soul element only as an inner coloring, an inner sensual feeling. Some of them migrated into the regions that earlier had been covered with ice. There they weaned themselves away from this inner sensual feeling and again strengthened their bodies. This is how Western civilization was added to that of the East. Even today, you can see from the glacial formation here on the mountain tops that the earth was once thoroughly frozen in this region, enabling the people who moved here to strengthen their bodies.

You also find reason for the decline of the Roman Empire in these things. This dates back to the age when Christianity was first beginning to spread. Yes, if Christianity had spread among the Romans, the result would have been pretty bad. The Romans, who possessed only the remnant of the oriental, Asian culture, had become so weakened that they could not accomplish anything. Then the people of the northern, ice-covered regions arrived with their more sturdy bodies, and the Roman Empire consequently perished. These northern people with their more sturdy bodies took over the cultural and spiritual life.

History describes this as the "barbarian" invasions, in which the Romans perished when the Germanic tribes arrived. These are really today's Europeans—the Germans, the French, and the English—because they are all basically Germanic people. The French have only absorbed a little more of the Roman element than the Germans for example. All this is based on the fact that these people came from regions where they could absorb the influences of the universe, whereas the other people with their wisdom lived only on the Earth. These people that came from the north renewed the whole civilization. So you see, this is how nature is related to everything that takes place in history.[14]

This long passage brings into focus another aspect of nutrition and therefore more choices for families to make. If a young family chooses consciously to live in a northern area where it is indeed more difficult to live and requires more energy—and living on top of the world we are closer to the stars in a way—how does this affect our lives, our children's lives? This kind of influence, which affected the northern people, is indeed a kind of nutrition, a cosmic nutrition in which we all partake. How does that develop the child?

I see many young couples choosing to live and have children in my small town. The children are beautiful and sturdy with bright eyes. I see them bundled up in their warm clothes on sleds, enjoying the winter wonderland. What effect does this have on these little beings? Do they become sturdier and have a definite future task like the Germanic tribes of former times? Or has that time passed?

What about the little ones who grow up in a city like New York, surrounded by cement, living on the 18th floor, hardly walking and feeling their legs, with only a park in which to experience a little bit of nature? There the park experience is an extra and not part of life; life is in the tall skyscrapers, cars, shopping trips, and entertainment venues that accompany such an artificial life. How does that influence children as they grow up increasingly separate from the

---

14 Steiner, *From Comets to Cocaine*, p. 283.

wonders of nature, mountains, brooks, wildlife, water, and mud? The child sees only manmade places such as museums, scientific settings that are separate from life itself. No wonder such great cities are homes to thousands of psychiatrists and psychologists whose offices are swamped with patients. Many of the children become out of sync with their inner nature. They never know who they are and they seek negative experiences to fulfill their lives. Young people's lives have become as meaningless as those of the adults who surround them. They run from one entertainment to another, never having any peace within themselves. From an early age, they never know what boredom is.

Boredom is healthy. It creates a space in which the person lives and thinks without requiring a filling up. The person feels the emptiness, does not fear it, but feels it. Then, somehow, some creative juice starts moving within the soul, and the person starts something they had not thought of before. Creativity enters. Artists are not always creating, but they have time when they need to do nothing and experience solitude, boredom. It is a painful state, but one that people need to go though so that they are not always living with the question, "What can I do to entertain myself?" like an open mouth saying, "Feed me."

In this state of constant entertainment, people become easy prey to the advertising industry. How can we suck up the energies of these young ones or older ones for profit? We find this, with sexual undertones, in the clothing industry, the computer game industry, the sports industry, the publishing industry and pretty books that contain only empty words, food that appeals only to taste and creates inner chaos, and much more.

In choosing a simpler setting for children to grow up in, one has to make sacrifices: smaller incomes, less sophistication and prestige. These decisions must be made by the family, together, and they require enormous strength, but if one has thought it out, then the family can benefit from either living in big cities or moving to rural areas. In big cities one can find some kind of healing by getting away and taking the children to mountains, seashores, camps, hikes, or stays on farms to work together growing food and experiencing the animals that provide us food. This, rather than spending time running around museums where the little ones develop big intellects and trade their beautiful red cheeks for pallid, weak little faces. Their muscles atrophy, as well, and in later life they will break bones and never enjoy a lively old age. Their sedentary city lives will have weakened them, and sclerotic diseases and other illnesses including early dementia may set in with untold suffering.

In cities, the senses are constantly assailed by outside stimulation that, as mentioned, preys on the little ones as well as on adults. They never have a minute alone and never develop their sacred space. There is no space, no inner space, because it is all filled, never giving inner peacefulness a chance. It is no wonder so many end up on a psychiatrist's couch. Untold psychological problems come to fruition in these settings, and by living in the city we set our children up for them.

> Humanity can very easily become aware of this moral and spiritual relationship to the plant-world by giving natural feeling free play. Human beings need the plants not only for food but also for their inner life, in order to nourish within themselves the feelings and experiences necessary for a life of soul. They need the impressions from the plant-world on the physical plane if their life of soul is to be fresh and healthy. That is something which cannot be over-emphasized. A deficiency in the human soul soon becomes apparent if it is shut off from the fresh, vitalizing influence of the plants. In a person who, through city life, is practically cut off from immediate contact with the plant-world, someone possessed of deeper insight will always perceive a certain inner deficiency. It is absolutely true that the soul suffers harm from the loss of the spontaneous joy and delight arising from direct contact with the plant-world. This loss is one of the shadow-sides of modern civilization to be found chiefly in great cities. We know that there are people who can

scarcely distinguish a grain of oat from a grain of wheat; yet to be able to do so belongs to a healthy human nature. This may be regarded as an indicative. One must view with regret any prospect of a future when humanity might be altogether deprived of any direct contact with the world of plants.[15]

This is why I always tell my city friends: Please move, for the sake of your children. Go to a smaller city or community. I feel much more invigorated living in the north, here in the cold climate, especially in the winter. In the south, far south, my body becomes lazier, less energetic, more likely to take it easy, eat a banana off the tree and relax, never mind about tomorrow. Here in the north there is no tomorrow if one does not work at keeping warm. One would simply die, so there is something valid about living in the north to become sturdier, more awake. I will discuss this topic again, the topic of cosmic nutrition, which, in the anthroposophical view of nutrition, is as important as physical substance intake. This is something totally new and foreign to the materialistic science of nutrition where, as quoted before, the body is seen as a combustion engine and food as its fuel.

In the mountains, everyone is nourished by living and simply being here. We breathe the fresh air, drink the pure glacial waters, spend time outside, look at the stars, cut wood to keep warm, live on very simple foods because that is all there is, sit by the fire, and spend plenty of time reading during the long nights. The children play outside, enjoy the cold, and are not separated from nature as are their little counterparts in the large cities.

I once invited a family from China to our farm in the Midwest. They had one son who was exceedingly bright. The family had always lived in Shanghai in tall buildings. This ten-year-old boy had never interacted with the country. He would not come out of the car for fear of the dog, and he could not walk around the garden

---

15   Steiner, *Macrocosm and Microcosm*, pp. 189–190.

because of the bees, butterflies, and other creatures that flew near him. He was afraid of so much life around him. I tried to have him touch the plants, the leaves, but he could not; it was too much life. Touching a little worm was out of the question. He had been completely weaned from nature and was intensely afraid. His domain was computers, which he loved along with other machines. He said he wanted to become a train expert, making time schedules and the like, dealing only with numbers and machines. Observing that particular child I was devastated, stunned, and felt terrible that his parents had helped in the development of such a little being. There seemed no life within his soul, and I wondered what would happen to him as an adult. He was an example of intellect-genius gone wild. How many of these little beings are born now in our world with no contact with nature whatsoever? To them food comes denatured in packages; machines surround them and only their fingers and their intellect get any exercise. Where are their feelings? Can they have feelings for others? Certainly not. Where are their souls? They are only intelligence, intellect. What if they become brilliant doctors or engineers? What will they invent? This is what we foster when we raise children in artificial settings. We create monsters rather than human beings.

This was an extreme case, but there exists all sorts in between. As responsible mothers and fathers, we must think about the implications of our choices. Yes, I love the city; it is a wonderful place, but is it the best place for a child? And how do we balance the negative forces with positive ones? Most people like their comfort zones, their selfish goals, and forget the hardship they impose on their families, whether it involves employment or a reluctance to give up a comfortable life in the city. If one knows the effect of such a lifestyle, then precautions can be taken to counteract the negative effects, so that the city life can be less harmful.

Because I had been brought up in the country, on the outskirts of cities, I chose to live in the country as soon as I was able to afford it. After having children there was only one choice, and that was living in the country. We did live on the outskirts of bigger cities for a few years, but every weekend we spent walking in beautiful national parks. When my son reached the age of ten he was full of energy, and sitting in school was difficult for him. So I looked in the local newspaper and found an old twenty-three-foot sailboat. We bought it and put it in at the Niagara Falls sailing club. There were at least fourteen knots of currents in that little harbor. Before we sailed my son and I took a rather difficult class in boating from the Great Lakes Coast Guard. We got our diplomas and in the spring went sailing. The first day was a challenge, as I had never really sailed a big boat, but we all took to it. Little by little we ventured into the large lake. My son picked it up quickly, and it was just what he needed, to be confronted with the danger of the elements: strong winds, currents, and the rocking boat. His sister was not too enthusiastic, but we were all excellent swimmers, so I never worried. Providing these challenges to that particular child saved me lots of headaches. He was fully engaged, happy, and could even as a small child be involved in something meaningful. Later he would not need to use drugs or drive fast cars; his needs had been met by nature's forces, by the elements, which demanded quick thinking, strength, courage, and responsibility.

I tell this story because parents will have to decide what it is they will provide to meet their child's needs. Mothers who listen to their children will know what they need, and they will provide it. The boat was not very expensive, so cost was not an issue in my case. Going for walks and hikes costs nothing, and bicycling, cross-country skiing, swimming, running, ice skating, gardening, owning a dog—or two depending on where one lives—are inexpensive activities.

In my case I was aware of who the child was that had been sent to me. When I was carrying my son I was living alone in the mountains of Vermont, in Robert Frost country. I had a small but beautiful rented chalet heated only by wood. I spent the last few months of my pregnancy living there alone amid beautiful pine trees and lots of snow. I had no energy whatsoever for reading my usual piles of books on philosophy, psychology, or religion. Instead I knitted lots of colorfully designed baby clothes and read all sorts of books about the sea. I could not get enough of them, one after another. I read Tristan Jones' sea adventures, as well as the poetry of Blake, while waiting for this child to be born. So I knew intuitively that this little being would love the sea, and now he is a fisherman in Alaska and Washington State and has just purchased his third boat. He is an accomplished tall-ship sea captain, as well as an engineer of boat systems, a musician, and a minstrel.

Because I had prepared myself for this birth, I knew who this little being was. He was coming to me from far in the past, and I was there to receive him and give him what he needed. I was a vegetarian and so was he. We were both extremely healthy. For the first three years of his life, his karma and mine did not allow him to be with his father.

This is just a small example for expectant mothers, to learn to be extremely attentive to who the little being is that is coming to them as if by magic. We must recover the sense of magic that happens when two beings meet and decide to have a child, or better, when the child has decided to come and is there for the two beings to accept. It might mean that the child will have only one parent, and that is also karma.

It might be that this child requires the mother to eat meat or perhaps not to eat meat. Many spiritual, religious traditions tell the young couple that they need to make their body as clean as they can for the welcoming of the child. This requires no immoderate drinking for at least a year, if not more, before conception, a life of quiet meditation even amidst the busy lifestyle of the city, cleanliness of habits, good natural foods, plenty of rest, good books to prepare for the child and to foster idealistic goals. Then the child to come will enter into this world in a nest of warmth and love, which is a great gift.

The same process applies to parents who decide to adopt children. They must make themselves ready for that child who has chosen them as parents through various magical channels—and the mother knows this.

> Someday, when people pay attention to what Anthroposophy says. Perhaps novels will even be published for pregnant women, and when pregnant women read them, they will receive impressions of ideal human beings. As a result, beautiful babies will be born who will grow to be strong, fine-looking human beings. What a woman does with her head during pregnancy becomes the source of what takes place in her womb. She shapes and forms the child with what she imagines, feels, and wills.[16]

During my first three months of pregnancy, which had been thoroughly planned, I left Iran and I went to Crete where I walked through the Santa Maria gorges and lived in my tent by the sea. I swam from the beautiful beaches by the mountainous shore, visited old abandoned monasteries, and ate wonderful food including thick creamy fresh yogurt and juicy peaches, and warmed myself under the great Sun. That was my gift to my son. I was alone and did not have much money, but I never felt abandoned. My son was getting everything he needed, even though I basically had no home or job, had left the child's father, and owned nearly nothing—except the beautiful sunshine, the starlit sky, the crystal clear sea, delicious food, interesting travelers, and a great trust in the future. I was never a worrier. This little being was coming, and I was living in the moment with not a care except to eat well, heal my body and soul from love's pain, enjoy the magical scenery of Greece, and wait until winter's gift was ready to come. Sometimes life gives us the best in the most unconventional, painful ways.

---

16 Steiner, *From Comets to Cocaine...*, p. 160.

This little story might appear to lead us astray into subjects that are not related to food, but actually we are going right into what real food is. What was I providing for this child even before he was born? Even though I loved the people dearly, I could not very well stay in a country torn by revolution, extremism, intolerance toward women, and incredible pain inflicted on its masses through a regime of terror. My son would have to be brought up in a clearer spiritual, political, social climate. Spending time in beautiful Crete and other islands of Greece among its architectural treasures was a beginning, a wonderful beginning for new life.

What was I providing for my son and myself we can call "cosmic nutrition." My body, soul, and spirit were exposed to the night skies, the stars, the elements, the sun, sand, artistic beauty, good foods, good company, and silence. I was feeding my twelve senses to the maximum.

Like human thoughts that have been rendered in works of art to be resurrected in the minds of those who see and understand them, universal thoughts celebrate resurrection in us when we approach nature's creation with open minds and senses. *This is the cosmic nutritive stream.* Impressions and perceptions of the world about us flow continuously into us through all our senses. This stream consists of formative forces, the same forces that come from the periphery of the cosmos and create the various plant species. They are the same forces that build the human organism and become its very flesh and blood. Our perceptive life is actually participation in the life of the whole universe, though we are no longer conscious of it. The world of nature spread out before our senses is the product of divine activity, the same activity that made our bodies. These bodies are actually microcosmic copies of the universe....

Today [we] are on our own in a godless world and must think and feel and will our groping way back to the creative forces of the universe as free spirits.

Human thinking, will, and feeling can, if we make the necessary effort, find the way to a new harmony with divine creative thinking, reexperiencing cosmic thoughts in full participation. Achieving this to some degree activates regenerative forces in our organisms. Failure to attain this leaves our thinking abstract and unreal, merely something made up by the brain, and has a disintegrating effect because we lack connection with the nourishing formative cosmic forces. People in this category like to talk about not having to bother with eating, and instead swallow a chemically equivalent few pills. Their ideal is to stay perfectly passive, to save time, to avoid coming to grips with Earth and cosmos in the ways required for adequate nourishment. Body and soul would both dry up, under such a regime; the body becomes sclerotic and the soul joyless and incapable of interest. The term *uplifting* suggests something of the element required. We all know how nourished we feel when we have entertained great thoughts or experienced the beauty and wisdom in art and nature. Some may even have noticed how little interest they feel in material food while on a mountain climb, especially up among the high peaks.[17]

The little child was growing slowly within me, and I had nothing to do with it. Something was working from far out there, and I am thankful that I had the intuition to give this child what he needed. I was helping the cosmic forces that were magically working within my belly to produce such a wonder. The whole zodiac was involved. I had chosen for this child to be born in February, in the sign of Aquarius like his father, and that region of the cosmos, its stars and planets, were doing their job. I had always loved to study philosophy, but now this—new life being created—was beyond all the mysteries.

The cosmos resounds. There is a twelvefold sounding from the zodiacal constellations, a sevenfold sounding from the planetary spheres.

The cosmic "Word," described by St. John as having "made everything that was made," draws the consonantal framework of its body from the zodiac, the sounding vowels of its all-permeating music from the planetary spheres.... Earth, like Heaven, is shaped by the musical ordering power of this cosmic Word, which reaches

---

17 Hauschka, *Nutrition*, pp. 28–29.

into matter itself and gives it patterns of coherence. Earth is the materialized "cosmic Word...the end of God's path."

When we go into nature and look at trees and flowers, stones and mountains, and veins of ore, trying to grasp all we see in a way that leads us toward the archetypes, perhaps here and there we can glimpse what lies beneath the surface. This means beginning to read the divine cosmic Word again—reading that frees it from captivity in matter.[18]

It is a great gift if the young mother is aware of all of this before she receives the child. The child will most definitely feel welcomed, after departing the spiritual world of great beings to enter the earthly world with all its darkness. It takes great courage to come to this Earth nowadays. Steiner always mentions that some great beings are waiting to come to this Earth, but the Earth is so materialistic that they cannot come yet. We are not ready for their gifts. It is time some young people make themselves ready for these new souls full of ideals and greatness to come and help our sorrowful state with their almighty light. I travel a lot, and I am constantly amazed at the small beings I meet in hidden towns around the world. Little beings with lovely intelligent eyes, ready to do their part if we do ours.

A person of high moral principles also needs parents who transmit a physical body suitable for the functions of those moral gifts. Thus, people have their parents and no others because they are unique individuals.

An individuality seeks the parents, though through the guidance of higher beings.... True knowledge, however, shows maternal love to be even more profound. It shows that this love is present before birth, even before conception, as a force that guided the child to that mother. The child loves the mother even before birth, and maternal love is the reciprocal force. Spiritually

---

18   Hauschka, *The Nature of Substance*, p. 232.

regarded, therefore, maternal love extends to the time before birth; it is rooted in mutual feelings of love.[19]

Now we will go further into this very complicated subject of nutrition as we, little by little, clarify the mysterious processes that go on within our very own bodies. We usually think that we are nourished by the food we take in. Simply put, as I said before, we put fuel into our organism and then we live. This is materialistic thinking: we take in fuel from some substance or other depending on where we happen to live, and then magically we grow, we live. But, as I have begun to reveal, we have other means of providing nourishment to the body. It is a fallacy to think in terms of substance that makes us live. A few passages below will shed some light on this complicated process. It will take, as usual, a bit more work from the reader to try and understand these processes; nothing is simple.

> We transform the surrounding world into concepts through our senses. That is to say, as our souls digest the world, soul content is embodied in us. In a less subtle kind of feeding on the world, we absorb its substances and transform them through physical digestion. Current nutritional physiology regards only the material process to be within its proper scope.[20]

> We compared the earthly nutritional stream with a plant growing from above downward, going through progressive etherization until it finally disappears through the intestinal wall and into the blood. The process of digestion subjects food in its original coarse form to a gradual breakdown. First, it is reduced mechanically by chewing, and then reduced chemically by passing through the stomach and intestinal tract. Carbohydrates are changed to sugars, fats to glycerine and fatty acids, with the result finally etherized into the spiritual microcosm through the intestinal

---

19 Steiner, *Rosicrucian Wisdom*, pp. 71–72.
20 Hauschka, *Nutrition*, p. 8.

wall. Just as the cosmos responds to the plant's etherization by producing seed, likewise human protein is precipitated on the far side of the intestinal wall.

We may ask: What constitutes the seed of this reversed plant? Earthly food goes in particular to nourish the nervous system. Observation in areas of starvation in Central Europe provide the necessary confirmation of this fact. Malnutrition shows itself first in nerve-sense degeneration, leading from the symptoms of forgetfulness, nervous depletion, inability to think, and so on to disturbed sight and hearing. Of course, the damage then spreads to the whole organism, since the whole nervous system is "trophic." We have to conceive the "seed" of the etherized stream of nutrients as consisting of the activity of the nerves and senses.

What does a seed do when planted in a fertile soil? It produces roots and a new plant. Our nerves and senses do the same thing. They reach out as roots into the universe to perceive and partake of the spiritual sustenance it offers as creative forces arising from divine thoughts, enabling a new "plant" to grow in us. That plant is reversed, too; it grows down from the spirit into matter, condensing its stream of suprasensory, non-material energy quite literally into flesh and blood.

It might be argued that some people seem to get along without a cosmic nutritional stream because they never give a thought to universal truth. Certainly, this may continue for some time and with no obvious evidence of severe illness and degeneration. This happens, however, only because no one is in fact wholly shut off from all participation in a larger life. It is true, too, that the quality of one's bodily substance is very different from that of a person who relates in a loving way to the surrounding world.[21]

Now we come to the more complicated aspect of nutrition as developed by the insight of Dr. Steiner in his course for doctors, as stated by Dr. Hauschka previously: "Earthly nutriments work mainly on the nerve-sense organs, whereas cosmic nutriments maintain the digestive organs, which are built by the blood. The

---

21 Ibid., p. 30.

metabolic organs consist of cosmic substance but serve the earthly nutritional stream; the nerve-sense system is made of earthly substance but serves cosmic nutrition."[22]

The whole of our organization is not formed and nourished by the food we take in through our mouths; rather, that food, as nutritional substance, goes only to the brain. The organism as a whole, for both animals and human beings, is formed and its hidden structure maintained by everything that comes to us as nourishment through our sensory organs....

Conversely, consider the description of the nerves that Rudolf Steiner provided for doctors and priests, for whom he describes the nervous system as a digestive organization. The ether, streaming in through our senses, carries light, sound, and life. It travels down through our nerves into our entire organization. We must imagine that one stream goes out into the world, and its ash nourishes the brain; the other stream goes down into the body, furnishing us with etheric substance. Steiner describes how we actually inhale warmth in our senses, and light, sound, and life are contained in that inhaled warmth. We also exhale this warmth, but not into the outer world. The exhaled warmth flows into our body. We inhale air and exhale warmth in our chest-organization, but the exhalation does not go out into the world, but down into our body. These two streams—the exhaled warmth that carries light, sound, and life, and the inhaled air— meet and finally settle in what science describes as lymph. This cosmic stream carries light, sound, and life as it descends, and when descending it leaves the light behind in the head, where it becomes our inner light. Sound is left behind to become the inner activity of our rhythmic system. Life goes right down into physical substance, and this is what really fills and nourishes us. The life ether takes hold of carbon, the sound unites with oxygen, and nitrogen and light work together with sulfur and phosphorus.[23]

---

22 Ibid., pp. 29–32.
23 König, *Earth and Man*, pp. 194, 252.

It is important to live with such pictures which counteract the materialistic views taught by contemporary science. Living into these pictures as much as we can will help us understand nutrition on a deeper level.

> I have often been told that it is shattering to learn that our eyes should be considered digestive organs. Why is this?... We realize that, to provide us with sensory impressions, our sensory organs must be digestive organs; to digest food, our liver, spleen, kidneys, and intestines must be sensory organs. There is no other possibility. How can they digest if they cannot sense what they are actually digesting?
>
> Dear friends, one of the great mysteries of science today is this: when you place a substance on your tongue, how do the salivary glands "know" exactly what kind of substance it is? The fluid they excrete changes according to the substance. Put a stone on the tongue, and nothing will flow, put meat on it, and a certain saliva will be produced; with cabbage, another kind of saliva is produced. But the mystery is solved when we realize that the salivary glands are not simply machines that secrete a certain amount of fluid. They secrete a particular sort of saliva, in fact, because they have tasted the nature of the substance on the tongue. In exactly the same way, our eyes "taste" the nature and the variety of colors; in tasting, the eye responds immediately by secreting, for instance, a certain amount of photopsin, with which it "digests" the color it has tasted. We see, but our eyes taste. We must learn to think of our sensory impressions as digestive processes and our nutritive and digestive process in terms of sensory impressions.
>
> To substitute nerve activities for sensory impressions, as is often done today, is nonsense of course. The nerves sense as little as bones do. The liver, dear friends, the spleen, the gall, or the kidneys can sense much more than your face can.[24]

The pictures provided need to be lived with again and meditated upon. People interested in going more deeply into these processes

---

24 Ibid., p. 233.

can learn more by studying the aforementioned texts. It is beyond the scope of this book to delve into this deeper, but let this serve as a beginning. These words of Rudolf Steiner provide a powerful meditation: "The metabolic organs consist of cosmic substance, but serve the earthly nutritional stream; the nerve-sense system is made of earthly substance but serves cosmic nutrition."[25] Then Christ's words become a very powerful nourishing meditation: "I am the way and the truth and the life" (John 14:6).

The birth of my second child, a daughter, was a very different experience than my son's planned birth. My daughter came when she wanted, unexpected. I was busy teaching Spanish in a Connecticut high school and became pregnant at Christmastime. I'd had a thought for many years—a daughter born in October—and that turned out to be her birth date. She came at a very busy time in my life. I was working as a full-time high school teacher, wife, and mother of a five-year-old. I taught all that year, feeling her kicks in my stomach, out of breath from talking all day.

During the spring I had to train my body because, before I became pregnant, I had planned a trip to South America, where I would hike the Inca Trail. I decided not to change my traveling plans, ignoring my obstetrician who said I was crazy. All spring I biked to school, even though my growing belly got a bit in the way. Six months into the pregnancy I left for Peru with a female coworker, while my husband took care of our son.

I decided that I would not carry my belongings, as that would be too much, so I hired two porters to carry and set up our tents, and off we went for one month of walking. I believed my daughter needed to be there, to experience this part of the world, so I called her my Inca princess as I walked every day in sumptuous majestic settings. We hiked on the old Inca trails, beautiful paths made of stone, climbing up and down mountainous terrains. We walked

---

25 Quoted in Hauschka, *Nutrition,* p. 32.

through old temples nestled high in hidden corners of the mountains. It was idyllic, and I hiked carefully, taking large breaths of magic air. After the hike we traveled through much of the Peruvian countryside all the way to Bolivia and Lake Titicaca, enjoying the delicious food cooked by people who lived in the region. That was my gift to this wonderful child. Again I was surrounded by mountains, flowing rivers, ancient architecture with mysterious temples hiding ancient knowledge of gods, temple priests, offerings, gold, and pools. I had plenty of fresh air, stupendous views, and clear skies. She was receiving what she needed.

She was born on my birthday, at 5:00 a.m., after I had worked until 10:00 the evening before attending parent–teacher conferences. That beautiful Persian-looking child, with dark eyes and hair, was extremely social. My act of teaching children all day during the entire pregnancy was also what she needed. She is not a country-loving child but loves the city, where she now lives in a metropolitan center in the Pacific Northwest. She thrives on people, people, and more people. She also has a great connection to the Spanish language. When she was fourteen, we traveled to Ecuador, because I wanted her to see South America. She was very comfortable among people wherever we traveled. I often allowed her to go to remote villages with friends we met who were her age, and she was never fearful. We went back again when she was sixteen, and when she was eighteen she went for three months to Patagonia on an Outward Bound trip and truly enjoyed the Pampa gaucho cowboys who were part of the experience there. She moved to Barcelona, Spain, for two years when she was nineteen and connected with many people.

She recently received a degree in psychology. She has friends, men and women, from all walks of life, races, nationalities, and ages. She is a modern child. You won't see her in the gardens looking at plants like her mother does, but in the busy city enjoying facescapes in the midst of people. The more faces the better.

Although I breast-fed my daughter, I had to extract the milk which her father then gave to her when I was away teaching, since he stayed home to study. I would run home for the 10:00 a.m. feeding, then again for lunch. We had moved into a basement apartment so I could be close to home (three minutes) for breast-feeding. It was an ugly place, but I had to work to provide for the family. One does not always have the opportunity to do the perfect thing, which would have been to stay home. I taught until she was one and a half, at which point she became ill with a very high fever. I attribute it to my teaching and having to get her up and take her to a baby-sitter for a few hours a day. But again, that is what I had to do out of necessity. I then quit the teaching job and stayed home to take care of the family, as my salary was then no longer needed.

I breast-fed both of my children for more than a year. It was extremely convenient, especially if they had some childhood illness. It calmed them down and provided the best nutrients. I was fortunate to have a lot of milk. In the animal realm the skinny cows have the most milk, more than the bigger cows, and the most cream as well. I was thin, so my kids were very healthy, and my milk provided plenty of fat for them—good fat, not bad.

For women who have a tendency to have less milk there are some wonderful foods which they can eat to increase their milk supply: almonds, oats, raisins, dates, and yogurt. These will automatically bring more milk to the mother. If the child cries a lot, the mother should stay away from onions, chocolate, coffee, and strong stimulants so as not to transfer them to the milk and make the child nervous or cranky. To decrease the milk when weaning the child, one should drink sage tea all day and it will dry up the milk supply.

Regarding nutrition, it must be understood that there is a spiritual bond between mother and child, especially during the early years; the mother who breast-feeds her child pays attention to this relationship. The milk contains more than its physical, chemical components; spiritually, it is related to the child. It is evident from spiritual research that the milk issues from the mother's etheric body. Because the child's own etheric body is not yet born, at first it can tolerate only what has been prepared by another ether body. Statistical evidence shows that, of those who die in infancy, 16 to 20 percent have been breast-fed by their own mother, whereas 26 to 30 percent have not. This is an indication of the close affinity between the ether bodies. The affinity expresses itself physically in family likeness. Traits and characteristics pointing to the line of descent develop and become established during the first years.[26]

A timeless yearning of the human race has been the "Promised Land, flowing with milk and honey." Nonetheless, it is based on a true vision of wholesome living that might deserve to be labeled "human." We would like to get to the bottom of this mystery.

Milk…is humanity's original and oldest food. It was manna from Heaven at the time when Earth's atmosphere…was permeated with a milk-like protein substance, the last remnant of which is our present-day nitrogen. This was the beginning of earthly human evolution. We started using the milk of our animals from the very beginning and have continued to do so ever since. We see that period of evolution repeated in each individual's infancy and childhood.

Milk prepares the body for habitation by the soul and spirit. It brings people down to earth and gives us a feeling for the oneness of humankind. We all breathe air that we own in common with everyone else. Perhaps, buried deep within us, there is the memory at work of having partaken in common of a cosmic milk, which still gives us a sense of social bond among individuals. Rudolf Steiner tells us that milk prepares human beings, in fact, to be creations of the Earth, without preventing us from being citizens both of the Earth and of the whole solar system. To go without milk would estrange us from the Earth and make us lose all connection with and feeling for humanity's earthly task. Therefore, Steiner says, we do well, even as adults, to let ourselves be gently tied down here by taking milk.[27]

---

26 Steiner, *Supersensible Knowledge*, p. 135.

27 Hauschka, *Nutrition*, p. 83.

When a child does not have the right milk, there are consequences:

> When you find that the liver of a fifty-year-old has hardened, the reason for this is usually (not always, but usually) that, as a baby, that person was fed the wrong kind of milk. Often what shows up as illness at the age of fifty was caused in very early childhood.[28]

Steiner then discusses how this hardening of the liver can cause cirrhosis of the liver and even cancer of the intestines or the stomach, because the liver is no longer able to distinguish what is good for the body. It is no longer the "inner organ of perception."

> Milk is the earliest of human foods. It is the product of living, sentient organisms, whose organs of lactation are part of the reproductive system. Reproduction is subject to Moon rhythms, the menses. Milk is therefore also connected with the Moon principle. It contains everything a growing organism needs and is a complete food, a liquid synthesis of protein, fat, carbohydrates, and mineral salts. All the building materials of the animal, vegetable, and mineral kingdoms are contained in milk as though in embryo.
>
> We may say, then, that ancient humanity lived chiefly on animal products. This form of nutrition dates back to the time before the Flood and continues as a source of human nutrition.
>
> According to what Spiritual Science has to tell us, milk is connected with the Moon principle, and...is part of the reproductive process. Spiritual Science reports that the Moon principle completely permeated the Earth in those ancient times when the two cosmic bodies were still a single entity. The atmosphere of this planet was suffused with a milky, egg-white-like substance which the totally different living creatures of the period absorbed as food. Only later, when the Moon separated from the Earth, did organs of lactation form inside the body as part of the reproductive system....
>
> Milk, then, is the original, earliest form of nourishment. We note that cattle, still held sacred in India today, have always played

---

28 Steiner, *From Crystals to Crocodiles...*, p. 53.

an important role in Indian mythology. It might be proper to call this phase "nutritional antiquity."[29]

A couple of years ago, I returned to India to work on a book on meditation (*Deliverance of the Spellbound God*) and I had a wonderful experience of the power that still lives in this "Mother of the Earth" country. I was sitting on some long steps on the banks of the Ganges that lead to a very old temple in Benares. A French lady had brought me there because it was her favorite temple, dedicated to a goddess. I sat next to a bubbly young woman selling little containers of milk so, like everyone else, I bought a couple of them to bring inside the temple as offerings. I carried the precious liquid inside the temple, which was dark and moist, impregnated with people's prayers, wishes, joys, and sufferings. Its walls blackened by time, it had an atmosphere thick with religious fervor. I was allowed inside this sweet-smelling cavernous old temple with its many dark niches. I followed the people and imitated them. They were helpful and showed me what to do. We reached the sacred center where the phallic statue stood, and there I gently splashed the milk. The statue was glistening with milk products and surrounded by gifts of flowers, plants, and various other offerings. We were nourishing the gods with the Earth's ancient food, milk, remnant of former wisdom that can still be encountered on the old continent. The Hindus had not been completely separated from this basic wisdom as in the West, where some women who are able to breast-feed now feel they do not need to nourish their little ones with perfect food because their breasts might not be so appealing afterward, even though there is no truth to that notion.

In that holy atmosphere, I plunged into the moon ambiance of primal nourishment that Steiner talks about in his book *Esoteric Science*. I also walked into the market streets and watched the milk

---

29 Hauschka, *Nutrition*, pp. 19–20.

brought into town in large containers on the backs of bicycles and small motorbikes, wrapped in icy cold burlap to keep it fresh. There was a line of housewives and some men coming to fetch their fresh milk to take home. Where I was staying they would have the milk blessed on altars dedicated to their favorite gods and then make sumptuous desserts with it for their family.

In the West nothing gets blessed. The denaturalized milk we buy at the store is no longer milk. We are slowly losing the right to even buy natural milk. There are court battles all around the country involving multinational companies that would like us, the people, to only buy *their* milk. Those same companies hire lawyers specifically for the purpose of taking small-scale farmers to court so they remain unseen by the public. No longer are we allowed to go to the farmer to buy our own milk, and farmers can be thrown in jail for selling milk to private customers. This is a reality in the Western world.

We no longer have primal nourishment, but a new poison. I always made sure my children had whole milk to drink that we brought directly from dairy farmers. I was very fortunate to live in areas where we could access a farming community in the form of community-supported agriculture where milk was available. After dropping the kids at school I would often spend time at the farm and watch the farmer milk the cows. We would chat, and I sometimes bottle-fed a calf or two. This is a cause for which young couples will have to fight if they want to preserve their right to eat what they want rather than what the big companies want to shove down their throats.

Now it is absolutely necessary to support a local farmer so that he or she can make ends meet each month. There is no other way but to work in solidarity. Farmers work hard and cannot worry about income; that is not their job. Their mission is to provide for the animals and gardens in their care. The rest is up to the people who eat their food. Therefore, part of our salary needs to go—must go—to the local farmer. That is the only way to stop the "industrial farming" monopoly that poisons the food supply for profit. I have lived in this way for twenty-five years. I was part of the first co-op when my son was born in Middlebury, Vermont.

It seems as if our society is bent on destroying what is fundamentally good and primal—milk itself. I suggest that the young mother and dad should find a nearby farm and go there; partake in milking the cows and feeling the warmth emanating from the huge cow stomach—a factory where mysteries not yet fathomed take place. Feel the warmth emanating from this cosmic being. Then, if you can still find a farm where the cow is allowed to graze, go into the field and watch the cows. Today, cows are shut up in large barns, where they never see grass; it is yet another attempt to kill the cows and prevent the milk from reaching people in its natural state. Young couples can get involved in their environment so that their children can survive and become whole human beings.

When I was a child I enjoyed cutting the milkweed and observing the milky liquid coming out of the stem, and I still do. In this magic moment, I always wondered where it came from. These plants are remnants of ancient plants that were part of the Earth in its infancy. Milk was a substance that was part of the thick atmosphere where the creatures breathed it in as nourishment.

As we evolve further, what will substitute for milk? If cows continue to receive their current inhumane treatment, the cow group soul might decide not to incarnate on Earth anymore. What will be the food of the future as the human body evolves?

When I was in my twenties I refused to have children or marry. I wanted to travel the world, and having children was not my goal. Staying home cooking, ironing, taking care of a husband were far from my mind. I wanted freedom to roam, study, read, walk, do sports; I was thoroughly selfish! But in my late twenties, during a forced holiday from my work in Tehran (I had to renew my visa), I was hiking in the Himalayas in western Nepal (my second trip there) among the rarefied clean air of ancient peaks, some over 26,000 feet

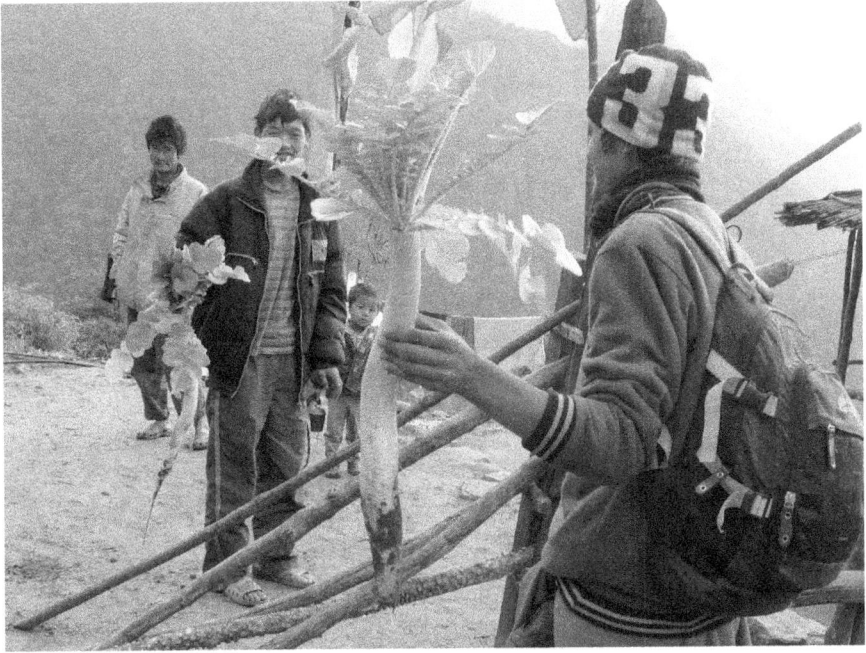

Daikon radish growing in a village in the Himalayas, Sikkim, India

high. There I made my decision that I would have children and show them the beauty of this Earth. I had at this time found their father, and perhaps I listened and felt that some little beings wanted me as their Mother and him as their Father. I said yes.

And now, as I have walked in many of this Earth's sacred paths, I marvel at the deep wisdom that is part of the different areas of the Earth. Each has its own culture, foods, animals, people, religion, architecture, geography, and each is very different from the other. That is what keeps me traveling to ever-distant places. Steiner says that when we die, we bring what we have done, experienced, and seen in this short life as a gift to the spiritual world, so I am determined to bring as much as I can, packed into this life.

Like the bees bring nectar from the flowers, we bring our own nectar in terms of our own experiences. The gods can't come to the Earth, but we humans bring them what we have lived through so

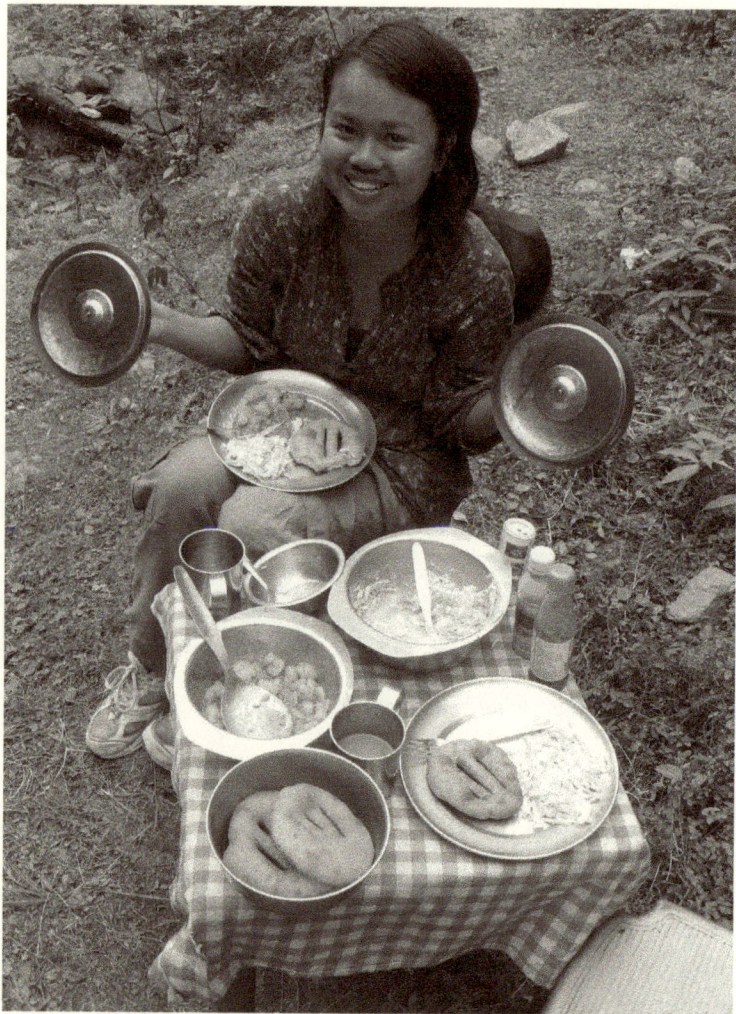

*Sikkim, India; a sumptuous lunch prepared by porters
on a trek behind Mount Everest*

they can know about it. I hope they won't be disappointed. I am doing my best.

Rudolf Steiner gives us this beautiful meditation addressed to our angel concerning our actions:

Just as what we have done in the past works on into our present life, the things we do in the present must work on into the future. But

54

this is possible only through the Angeloi, who direct their gaze to a person's present actions and bring them to fruition in the future....

When people perform some action, they should think of their angels saying inwardly, "May my Guardian Spirit receive this my act as a root and bring forth fruit from it." The more definite and vivid the imagery used when a person addresses his or her angel in connection with acts that should bear fruit, the more abundant that fruit can be in the future.[30]

This is one reason for writing this book—so that young couples, or young people and old (it is never too late), can do their best through their actions.

Now back to questions: How does geography relate to religion? Why are the Arabs in the desert and not near the Pacific? Why do dates grow in an oasis? Why the fat-tailed sheep? Why Moses on Mt. Sinai? Why "salt of the earth"? Why Hindus in India with their hot spices, vegetarian foods, and roaming cows? Why Native Americans in North America? Why corn in the Americas? Why Christianity in Ireland among the Irish monks? Why potatoes and oats in Ireland? Why Egypt, pyramids, and perfumes? Why China and Confucius? Why Japan and Buddhist temples in the Far East? Why tofu? Why rice? Why the white, yellow, copper, and black races? Why the Incas and their temples in South America? Why beans and corn and yams? Why Andalucía with its Arab, Jewish, and Christian cultures? Why olive trees?

Such questions might seem childish, but behind them is human evolution. I had these questions in my mind ever since I took up my travels or, actually, ever since I was a child marveling at the Arab language and culture into which I had been thrown. I was born with questions; they just come out of my mouth—why this and why that? I was seeking Mystery knowledge, which Anthroposophy offers. I am fascinated by these questions that seemed to

---

30 Steiner, *Karmic Relationships*, vol. 6, p. 55.

have no answers, but after being on the road all my life, some of them are being answered in a most amazing way. This is thanks to the study of Spiritual Science and the many lecture cycles given by Rudolf Steiner, which shed light on some of these mysteries. In all of these questions there is something about food hidden. All people eat; we eat what is available to us in where we live, and something comes to light when we concentrate on this aspect when traveling.

This fascinating area of food, people, customs, and geography is what we speak about in this book. Rudolf Steiner gives much food for thought to help us begin this world journey.

> Originally, different races lived in different regions of the Earth. One race developed in one region, another race in another. Why was this? It is quite correct to say that one planet has a particularly strong influence upon one part of the Earth, another planet upon another part. In Asia, for instance, the land is strongly affected by what streams to the Earth from Venus—Venus the evening star. What streams from Saturn works with particular strength upon American soil. And Mars works particularly strongly upon Africa. So we find that each of the planets works particularly strongly upon some specific part of the Earth. They radiate their light from the various places where they stand in the heavens. The light of Venus, for instance, works quite differently upon the Earth than does the light of Mercury. This is connected with the different formations of mountains, of rocks. Thus the different races inhabiting different regions of the Earth are dependent upon the fact that one part of the Earth is particularly receptive to the influences of Venus, another part to the influences of Saturn, and so on.[31]

I will mention a few countries and some of the food that is eaten in those areas. I chose a few items for specific reasons, so it is not a complete description of the diets in these countries, nor is it meant

---

31 Steiner, *From Sunspots to Strawberries...*, p. 139.

to be. Diets encompass all sorts of mysteries and comprise an enormously complex topic, but such challenges have never stopped me before. Nevertheless, it is hard to know where to begin, so I will do so in a simple way by talking about salt and sugar.

Part 2: Mother Earth—
Her Food, Her People

The Far East, China

If you like Chinese food you will notice there is not much sugar in it, so it seems saltier in that respect. Saltiness is part of this diet rather than sweetness. Noodle soup is a common food which I loved when I was in Bangkok, Thailand, getting much of my diet from street vendors. I have since cooked many such meals for my family, and I still enjoy them when I am alone here in the mountains. I love a good salty soup with ginger, garlic, veggies, and noodles, especially after spending the day in the icy cold, skiing on steep slopes. Getting minerals through lots of vegetables and using much less sugar is very much part of the diet of the Far East. Young couples who adopt children of the Far East have to consider that these children will need a different diet from a Western one, and they must see to it that these children have their ration of rice, noodles, and lots of vegetables in order to be healthy and unburdened by the heavier diet of the Western world. What is hidden in this diet which comes from the Far East and its people? Steiner talks about that area of the world:

> We have to imagine that there was formerly solid ground where the Atlantic Ocean is today. We have Asia on the one hand [pointing to a map], the Black Sea here, below is Africa, then Russia and Asia itself. On the other hand, there is England, Ireland, and over

there also America. Formerly, everything in between was land, and here very little land; over here in Europe at that time there was actually a very large sea. These countries were all in the sea, and when we come up to the north, Siberia was sea, too; it was still all sea. Below, where India is today, the land rose a little above the sea. Thus we actually have some land there and land on this side, too. Where we find the Asian peoples today, the inhabitants of the Near East and those of Europe, there was sea—the land rising up only later. The land, however, went much farther, continuing right on to the Pacific Ocean, where today there are so many islands— Java, Sumatra, and so on; they were all part of the continent that used to be there—this whole archipelago. Thus, where the Pacific Ocean is now, there was a great deal of land with sea between the two landmasses.

The first peoples we are able to investigate remained in this region, here, where the land was preserved. When we look around us in Europe we can really say: ten, twelve, or fifteen thousand years ago the earth, the ground, became sufficiently firm for human beings to live on it. Before that, only marine animals were present, which developed out of the sea, and so on. If at that time one had looked for human beings, they would have been where the Atlantic Ocean is today. But over in eastern Asia, there were also human beings more than ten thousand years ago. Those people left descendants, of course, who are very interesting because of their culture, the most ancient on Earth. Today they are the Japanese and Chinese. They are very interesting because they are the last traces...of the oldest inhabitants of the Earth.[1]

The Far East has an ethereal landscape as can be seen in beautiful, elegant paintings with ephemeral, primal black ink brush strokes portraying a landscape of high peaks and light clouds, a floating landscape where nothing is really rooted on Earth but still belongs to the heavens. This is the home of rice growing, which reflects the quality of the surroundings. When we examine the rice grain we see radiating polygons and no center. It has grown under

---

1   Steiner, *From Sunspots to Strawberries...*, pp. 62–63.

cosmic influence and not under the strong influence of the Earth. It is not an earthy grain, but a cosmic one, full of light. It requires much swampy land to grow in, and it developed out of such lands.

When one eats rice, digestion is not encumbered by heaviness. On the contrary, it is light, as are the people of the Far East. They are ephemeral like the landscape, with fine, small features. A diet of potatoes certainly does not fit in with the Eastern diet. This diet often involves small game birds, ducks, eggs, and chickens, animals which reflect this atmosphere of light. In that part of the world, the bird family was more part of the ethereal scenery than were the cows and other ruminants. Birds live in the air, and rice is an airy grain full of light. So we can say that the Chinese have an airy light quality to their character.

Steiner mentions in many of his lectures that the Chinese people are descendants of Atlantis, the former continent which existed between the Americas and Europe. They are the remnants of that race, while Westerners are the beginning of another race. The Chinese language is a pictorial language infinitely more complex than the Western languages. The wisdom and culture of the Far East has not been surpassed. It achieved an advanced culture while the West was still living in barbaric conditions. But Steiner mentioned that those in the East had reached a perfect stage and have no more to achieve. Therefore it is up to the West, although highly imperfect and barbarous (to the Easterners), to achieve some new culture in spite of its imperfection. It was to reach toward something new. When one is perfect, then that is *it*. Imperfect means you can always improve.

China, as the rest of the Far East, still has a diet which stems from initiation knowledge, meaning its way of cooking is still full of wisdom. People there have not lost their ways yet, and their cooking still has remnants of deep knowledge. The food is presented in an ordered manner, different types of food for different purposes. For example, a soup is given to whet the appetite and start the digestive juices, as is warm tea. At a meal, one is given steamed food, stir-fried food, broiled food, some raw foods, pickled foods, very few sweets. Each food is meant to act on our different bodies: our physical bodies, our body of life (ether, in common with plants), our feeling body (astral, in common with animals), and our I. Such knowledge was instinctive in the older cultures, but now we have lost it and we need to regain it through our own efforts. In China it is still alive and if we study it with some insights brought from Spiritual Science, we can gain much.

So if we look at the Earth from out in space, light seems to be the dominant aspect in China and the whole Far East—light, rice grain, small birds. This can be seen even in the architecture, especially in the beautiful temples with their roofs turned up as if to be still part of the heavens—which it is, as China is not yet strongly incarnated. Its people have not arrived on Mother Earth, and they need light food so as not to feel so heavy. They are, in a way, lightly touching the ground. A diet based on Chinese food will bring lightness to the body and will allow for easier digestion. Let us look at this more deeply.

> The potassium content of rice is especially low...almost the same as cow's milk...; rice contains six times less potassium than European grains (wheat, rye, barley), ten to twenty times less than potatoes....
>
> Potassium and sodium have a polar relationship in the cell and tissue fluids of the organism. Thus, a high intake of potassium necessitates a high intake of sodium, so a diet rich in potatoes usually results in a high consumption of table salt....
>
> Rice, on the other hand, needs only very little salt. It is thus especially suited to a low-salt diet. Among the rice-eating peoples of the Far East, there is a conspicuously small desire for salt; hence the development of earthly forces is hindered. At the same time, the high phosphorus content of rice provides a basis for the development of spiritual forces.

Brown rice not only has importance in our diet but becomes an equal member of the spectrum of the seven grains. Its great advantages are its easy digestibility and its ability to unburden the kidneys and circulatory system.... The relatively low potassium content of whole-grain rice is important here for its water-reducing and "unburdening" qualities.[2]

Salt is food for thought. Minerals, salt included, is needed for thinking. Steiner often shows us the picture of the plant and references the human being as an inverted plant: the flower grows toward the light, the Sun, exposing its center. The roots grow toward the center of the Earth in darkness, and the leaves in the middle are the balance between Heaven and Earth and make starches. The roots draw the minerals up from the earth, and the minerals then travel upward and encounter carbon from the air in the magic of the leaf factories, where they then make carbohydrates (carbon united with hydrogen and oxygen, light processes, starches, and minerals), and then they go upward and disappear "magically" into blossoms, providing scents, oils, and seeds.

We have our head, with the nerves and brain like a tree, which needs the salty minerals for functioning. Our lower part, the metabolic system, the reproductive organs tend toward the Earth like flowers, and the middle part, with the breathing system and blood circulation, is like the leaves.

So here is a simple formula that one can start working with in cooperation with the plants.

Roots	nerve sense system	brain
Foliage	rhythmic system	lungs
Blossoms	metabolic and excretion	kidneys
Fruit	circulatory system	blood
Seed	organ formation	heart

---

2   Schmidt, *The Essentials of Nutrition*, pp. 231–232.

If you have a garden, begin to think in terms of the plants and their wonderful healing qualities—the roots, the leaves, the fruits, the seeds—feel their effects, feel what they have gathered and what it means to eat a fruit, or a salad, or a carrot. Live with color, what it has gathered from the Sun, and look at the root's color and form and the broad leaves of kale or spinach. Work with these pictures. Roots have a lot of salts, minerals, and that is good for the brain and thinking. Foliage is good for the lungs, so if you have a weak lung system, eat plenty of greens.

> The rhythmic system is the seat of healing forces in the organism, for its function is that of a balancer and harmonizer. Green vegetables stimulate and strengthen these forces, and therefore make especially wholesome foods....
>
> Blossoms act to stimulate human excretory functions. They drive warmth processes outward toward the periphery and dissolve and sweep away congested heat.... They affect mainly the kidneys, which are themselves, in a sense, blossoms become organs.[3]

Now we come to fruits.

> Fruits are not produced in direct continuation of the blossoming process, but the result of an answering cosmic radiation. Cosmic warmth and light form fruits and ripen them.... There is a parallel in human beings to this marvelous reversal from dematerialization in the blossom to the creation of fruit substances.... The creation of human tissue in the blood is a complicated interplay of earthly and universal forces, of which the fruit is an image.... We may therefore expect fruit to affect far more than just the intestinal functions; it also works on the circulation of human bodily fluids. A sufficient quantity of fruits in the diet therefore stimulates blood and tissue building in a way that keeps the body "fluid" in the broadest sense, as well as permeable by cosmic forces.[4]

---

3   Hauschka, *Nutrition*, pp. 78, 80.

4   Ibid., pp. 80–81.

Now the seed:

> Fruit tissue is related to the seed in the same way that circulation is related to the heart....
>
> All the four cosmic forces, or energies, are concentrated in the seed—light and warmth in oil and starches; formative forces and chemism in salts and proteins.... Seeds generally have a warming, nourishing, and "heartening" effect.[5]

Here we can say that seeds are good food for the heart and for the formation of organs. With these simple but profound insights, one can begin to live into the healing aspects of plants.

Let us return to our discussion of minerals, salts, and their complex functions.

> When plants are burned, they leave mineral residues in the form of ash.... Potassium, phosphorus, calcium, silica, magnesia, and sulfur are always predominant. Small amounts of aluminium, sodium, and chlorine are also present.... Some plants contain rarer elements; there is lithium in tobacco, iodine in seaweed and lichen, and titanium in roses.[6]

> Apart from the use of rock crystals, people today depend on the ability of plants to absorb minerals. Since the plant learned to root itself in the earth, its organization not only developed these organs for the earth, whereby the roots themselves are enriched, but also the flow of sap in the plant dissolves the minerals in a fluid element and carries them to the entire plant organization. In this way, they are connected to the proteins and accompany the other nutrients. The root itself, as the salt pole, is associated with that human system that is itself most mineralized...that is, the head and nerve-sense organization. This explains why rock salt is indispensable for forming thoughts.[7]

---

5   Ibid., p. 81.

6   Hauschka, *The Nature of Substance*, p. 118.

7   Schmidt, *The Essentials of Nutrition*, p. 210.

❀

Now we will speak more about rice and the Far Eastern diet. We can rightly see that in that part of the world we would find a people giving much nourishment to their upper pole, and thinking would be more developed in people there than elsewhere. The diet also includes many greens, vegetables, and roots, so the body is balanced, but it tends toward the head-thinking pole, so here we find nations of excellent thinkers. Through the use of rice, the thinker in the human being is developed.

This upper pole—our head system, our thinking thoughts—brings wisdom. We can easily see Far Eastern wisdom for ourselves. Its exquisite architecture and sculpture are unsurpassable. China's incredible musicians are masters. The magical dexterity of the Far Eastern people is a true wonder.

Now that we understand somewhat root-salt-nerve-thinking, we will have a look at phosphorus, one important mineral that is contained in rice. It is a long quote, but necessary to understanding the forces behind this substance, to meet the phosphorus being that is at home in rice.

In contrast to clay, phosphorus (or phosphate rock) is thinly scattered through the Earth's crust, like spices in a cake, instead of filling up whole regions, valleys, and basins.

> Phosphorus is everywhere in minute quantities.... If we place a piece of phosphorus on a plate, all sorts of interesting things can be observed. One is how the piece shines with a peculiar greenish glow in the dark. At the same time we notice a strange characteristic odor, exactly like that given off by a shower of electric sparks. This is caused by the formation of ozone. Phosphorus has the same capacity as electricity to condense oxygen in the air into ozone.
>
> Finally, we see fumes spiraling around the phosphorus. It does not look as though they were generated by it, but more as though they were encircling in toward it as a center, closing in on it. Suddenly the phosphorus ignites with a brilliant white flash

of spontaneous combustion, making a spurting, hissing sound—*ffffffffffffftt*—as it bursts into flame.

Phosphorus, then, shines and pours out light, but is also a condensing agent.... Our bodies contain a very considerable amount of material phosphorus. Nerves are built of protein high in phosphorous. Indeed the nervous system as a whole is as clear a revelation of the phosphorus.... Phosphorus flames give light, but are cold. Our nervous system endows us with the cool, clear light of consciousness.... It is to phosphorus that we owe awareness of our bodies and a bodily consciousness of selfhood....

The nerves with their phosphorus content—a substance known to chemistry as *nucleoprotein,* composed of lecithin and cholesterol—are at an intermediate stage of calcification. In a person tending to sclerosis, the walls of the blood vessels are coated with cholesterol and similar substances. As the disease progresses, these deposits calcify and bring on hardening of the arteries.

These facts indicate both the cause of sclerosis and the means of preventing it. The cause lies in a one-sided development of the phosphorus process with insufficient circulation to oppose it. The result of too-great intellectuality and self-centeredness is physical hardening in later life.[8]

By looking deeply at substances within the food, we can understand how rice will foster thinking through its phosphorus content putting its stamp on a whole people in the Far East and beyond: China, Japan, Korea, Iran, Iraq, Afghanistan, Pakistan and the other "stan" countries (Tajikistan, Turkmenistan, etc.), India, and Spain.

I view China as a father—Father China—an ancient father of the Earth, with its patriarchal system still in place, as opposed to India, which I see as Mother India, mother of religions. We in the Western part of the world approach the brothers and sisters realm, or at least we try.

If we look at a world map, we have Mother India on one side of the tallest mountains and Father China on the other, two huge

---

8   Hauschka, *The Nature of Substance*, pp. 135–137.

continents with the highest birthrates in the world and still growing. With global changes, China's consumption of sweets and table salts, plus a trend toward a Western diet, will bring enormous changes to that continent. They are quickly catching up to and surpassing the Western world, and positive and negative trends will follow. Incarnating more, the people of the Far East will not be content with their patriarchal system, but will demand freedom and individuality. In the same way, new trends in the Western world involving Eastern diets also bring changes in the other direction. The Far Eastern world will become more earthly and materialistic as its diet begins to include more meat, potatoes, and salt. The Western world, by adopting the Eastern diet of rice, soy beans, or total vegetarianism or veganism (which are becoming a bit of a sect), will become more "heavenly" and in some respects "lost in the clouds" and ungrounded. That will make it easier for dictatorships to rule those with their heads in the clouds, such as in Arizona's desert New Age mecca of Sedona, or California with its health fads. Here in the West people lose themselves in notions of "eternal beauty" of looks, fitness, and yoga and exiting the earth to attain Nirvanic never-never lands of peace. Meanwhile, shrewd politicians are having a field day with words of democracy and peace while creating wars and inventing new killing machines. They make billions doing it while many sleep on their yoga mats or chant about peace. Politicians see dollar signs for their meditation. I will bring up these topics again as we travel the world.

THE NORTH AMERICAN CONTINENT

From the Far-East diet that is lighter, rich in minerals and vegetables, rich, and less sweet, we will go to the opposite extreme, the West and its sweet tooth, meat and potatoes, excess salt, corn, milk, and peanut-butter sandwiches. The North American continent is the home of the American Indian Nation with its amazing gifts. In some areas one still has a feeling for the spirit of the Native American Indians who lived with nature.

> Native Americans descended from ancient times...and spoke of the "Great Spirit" ruling everywhere, ruling in everything. This Great Spirit was venerated particularly by human beings living during Atlantean times, when there was still land between Europe and America; the Indians retained their veneration and knew nothing as yet of intellect.[9]

One of the gifts of Native Americans is our Thanksgiving holiday, which began with the New England fall harvest. European settlers would not have survived without the gifts of the region's original inhabitants, which included corn, sweet potatoes, yams, and wild turkeys. The conquest of the far north would not have been possible had it not been for trappers, adventurers, and scientists who married native women, who fed and clothed them, gave them children, taught them survival skills, and accepted them into their tribes and communities. They learned to use various roots, berries, moss, and lichen and to dry the meat, hunt, fish, build homes, and make clothes. This continent actually owes everything to Native Americans. Not been much gratitude has been shown for their contributions, even on Thanksgiving Day.

This vast American continent is the former home of vast herds of bison (often called buffalo), a remnant of far more ancient beasts. This enormously powerful animal's manure is responsible for the rich black earth of the Midwest. Now cattle have replaced them. Here we enter the land of giants—giant landscapes, vast prairies, tall grasses, pines trees, oak savannahs, mountain ranges, and ancient rocks. It is the home of the corn grain, a beautiful golden seed, large and sunny, the starch on which much of the American food supply is reliant.

---

9   Steiner, *From Sunspots to Strawberries...*, p. 127.

A whole industry is built on it—corn syrup sweetener, corn starch, mush, corn meal, corn on the cob, corn muffins, corn cakes, fattening feed for cattle, pigs, and chickens, and don't forget ethanol to fuel cars. We can compare the large ear of corn to the tiny grain of rice. The Americas are the land of the corn and the potato.

In diners across the United States one sees a common meal of beef steak, huge baked potato covered with sour cream or cheese, green beans and corn, a salad, apple pie with ice cream on top, and of course a soda full of sugar, usually diet soda. The result is a body that is overweight and not prone to too much thinking because the stomach is too busy digesting. It personifies sluggish digestion and heart problems in the making. This is the opposite of the ethereal landscape, where cosmic forces prevail. Here we see earthy forces—forces that come from a center and radiate out to the self, self-centeredness.

Rudolf Steiner lets us know from his spiritual scientific findings that the American continent in many several thousand years will become the center of selfishness, just like China became a center of the highest wisdom so many thousands of years ago. Let us explore the potato, meat, corn, and milk diet and see how it affects the continent of North America.

The aspect which strikes foreigners when they land in North America is of course the largeness of it all, the abundance, the activity, and the initiatives. It is an industrious nation high in creativity: new cars, machines, technology, buildings, homes, and farms. We have it all, produced by seemingly relentless activity. But we also have the couch potato—very appropriate for our discussion.

> If we compare a potato to a carrot—first of all it appears quite different. Of course, the potato plant has a green part, and then it has the part we eat, which we call the *tubers,* deeper in the earth. If we think superficially, we could say that the tubers are the roots, but that is not correct; they are not roots. If you look down carefully into the soil, you can see the real roots hanging

off the tubers.... When we eat a potato, we are really eating a piece of swollen, enlarged stem...it is stem, or metamorphosed foliage. The potato is down there between the root and the stem. Therefore it does not have as much mineral content as the carrot does; it is not as earthy. It grows in the earth, but it is not related as strongly to the earth. In addition, it contains carbohydrates in particular—not so many minerals, but carbohydrates....

When we eat potatoes, first they go into the mouth and stomach, where the body has to exert energy to extract starch from them. Then the digestive process continues in the intestines. So that something can go into the blood and reach the head, there must be still more exertion, because sugar has to be made from the starch. Only then can it go to the head. Thus, we have to use even greater forces. Now consider this:... when I exert my strength upon something external, I become weaker. This is really a secret of human physiology—that is, if I chop wood, I use my external bodily strength and become weaker; but if I exert an inner strength, transforming carbohydrates into starch and starch into sugar, I become stronger. Precisely, through the fact that I permeate myself with sugar by eating potatoes, I become stronger. When I use my strength externally, I become weaker; if I use it internally, I become stronger. Therefore, it is not a matter of simply filling ourselves with food, but that the food generates strength in our body.... [The potato] requires a great deal of strength, but it leaves a person weaker afterward and does not provide a person with continuing strength....

Now, to the same extent that the potato is a rather poor food, all the grains—wheat, rye, and so on—are good foods. Grains also contain carbohydrates, and of such a nature that human beings form starch and sugar in the healthiest possible way. In fact, the carbohydrates from grains can make people stronger than they can make themselves by other means. Just consider for a moment how strong the people are who live on farms, simply through the fact that they eat large quantities of their own homemade bread that contains the grain from their fields. They just need to have healthy bodies to start with, then if they can digest the rather coarse bread, it is really the healthiest food for them. First, they must have healthy bodies, and then they become even stronger through the process of making starch and sugar.

The potato does little to care for the lung and heart. It reaches the head, but only, as I have said, the lower head, not the upper head. It does go into the lower head, where we think and exercise critical faculties. Therefore, you can see that, in earlier times, there were fewer journalists. There was no printing industry yet. Consider the amount of thought expended daily in this world today just to produce newspapers.... People who eat potatoes are constantly stimulated to think. They cannot do anything but think. That is why their lungs and heart become weak. Tuberculosis of the lungs did not become widespread until the potato diet was introduced, and the weakest human beings are those who live in areas where almost nothing is grown but potatoes—places where people live on potatoes.

But now what about potatoes? Suppose a scientist or a doctor were asked to say what effect potatoes have when they are eaten. As you know, potatoes have become a staple. In some places it is very difficult to dissuade people from feeding almost exclusively on them. What does modern science do when testing potatoes for their nutrition value? Laboratory investigations find what substances are contained in the potato. We find carbohydrates which consist of carbon, oxygen, and hydrogen in definite proportions; we also discover that in the human body these substances are finally transformed into a kind of sugar. But science goes no further than that.... If some animal is fed on milk, it may thrive. But if the milk is analyzed for its chemical components and if these chemical components are given to the animal instead of the milk, it will waste away for lack of nourishment. Why is that? It is because something is working in the milk in addition to chemical components. And in the potato, too, there is something more than the mere chemical components; there is the spiritual element. A spiritual element works everywhere, in all of nature.

If in Spiritual Science... genuine investigation is made into how the potato nourishes the human being, the potato is found to be something that is not completely digested by the digestive organs, but it passes into the head through the lymph glands, through the blood, in such a way that the head itself must also serve as a digestive organ for the potato. When potatoes are eaten in large quantities, the head becomes a kind of stomach and also digests.

There is a very great difference between eating potatoes and, for instance, good, wholesome bread. When wholesome bread is eaten, the material part of the rye or wheat is digested properly and healthily by the digestive tract. And consequently only what is spiritual in the rye or wheat comes into the head, where it belongs....

When things are genuinely investigated with respect to their spiritual quality, it becomes apparent that in this modern age humanity has been seriously injured by an excessive consumption of potatoes. Spiritual Science finds that eating potatoes has played a very large part in the general deterioration of health in recent centuries.

People believe that when their stomach is full of potatoes they have had a nourishing meal. The truth is that the health of their head is impaired, because the head itself then has to become a digestive organ.[10]

More on the potato:

Human beings, having one-sidedly developed only their brain, can think with great subtlety but are terribly clumsy fellows. It is important for the human being that not too much of the brain should be transformed. If too much has been transformed, a person may be a good poet but certainly not a good mechanic. This person will have no knack for doing things in the outside world....

Many people, owing to excessive consumption of potatoes, have transformed a very large part of their brain. The result is that such people are clever but unskillful. That is so often true today. They have to struggle to do things that they should really be able to do quite easily. For instance, there are people who are quite unable to sew on a trouser-button.... This is because the nerves which are nerves of perception in the more delicate organs have been transformed almost entirely into brain-nerves.

10   Ibid., pp. 86–88, 200–201, 105, 211.

Once I knew a man who had a terrible dread of the future. He argued that in olden times people's senses were more delicate, more keen, just because they had less brain, and that in the course of human evolution what had in earlier times belonged to the senses and enhanced their perception was metamorphosed into a clever brain. The man was afraid that this would go further, that more and more of the sensory brain would become thinking brain, so that finally human beings would be utterly incapacitated, going about with defective eyes and so forth. In olden times people went through life with good sight; now they need glasses. Their sense of smell is not nearly as keen as it was once. Their hands are becoming clumsy. And anything that becomes clumsy is bound to deteriorate. This man was afraid that everything would be transformed into brain and that the human head would get bigger and bigger and the legs smaller and smaller and all would atrophy. He thought quite seriously that human beings would someday be no more than round heads rolling around the world....

And his idea was perfectly correct. For if human beings do not find their way again to what they were once able to grasp through imagination, if they do not return to the spirit, then they will indeed become a round sphere of this kind! It is literally true that Spiritual Science does not simply make us clever. As a matter of fact, if we take it merely as one more theory, far from becoming more clever, we will become definitely more stupid....

Think of adults with a child before them. The adults may be a bit conceited about their own cleverness; if so, the child will seem stupid. But if the adults have any sense for what comes from the child's very nature, they will regard that as having far higher value than their own cleverness. One cannot grasp what exists in nature by brain work alone, but by being able to penetrate into the secrets of nature. Cleverness does not necessarily lead to knowledge. A clever person is not necessarily very wise. Clever people can't, of course, be stupid, but they may certainly lack wisdom; they may have no real knowledge of the world. Cleverness can be used in all sorts of ways: to classify plants and minerals, to make chemical compounds, to vote, to play dominoes and chess, to speculate on the Stock Exchange. The cleverness by which people cheat on the Stock Exchange is the same cleverness that one uses to study chemistry....

Obviously, too much should not be transformed into brain. If one were to dissect the heads of great financial magnates, one would find extraordinary brains. In this area, anatomy has brought a great deal to light. It has been possible to see proof of cleverness in a brain—but never proof of knowledge![11]

I quoted this because it is important to distinguish among the concepts *intellect, intelligence,* and *knowledge.* This is expressed masterfully by Rudolf Steiner, who makes it absolutely clear what a diet of potato fosters.

Now let us examine the meat diet and its impact. Along with cattle come milk products. The American people love their milk, drinking it and eating ice cream and cheese products, unlike the Eastern people who have no milk in their original diet. There milk is not part of the culture at all except for the nomadic tribes, former Huns of the steppe. In far western China, Mongolia, milk from horses and yak was part of the diet. This is true in all the countries surrounding the Caspian Sea where people are descendants of the Turks. Milk, as we have discussed, is a food which has a balancing effect on the human being. Steiner says that it gently roots a person to the Earth. We become earthly beings through our intake of milk as opposed to cosmic beings, meaning beings not too grounded. "Airhead" is a common expression depicting this trait. A strictly vegetarian or vegan diet will make a person more flighty and not rooted. Milk gives us roots. We live on Earth, not in the clouds, and we can see this in the American psyche. The good nature and willingness to help a neighbor, and perhaps a bit of naivety or childishness that Europeans detect in Americans, I think is the milk talking.

---

11   Ibid., pp. 143–145.

I am reminded of tall, strong young men and women who look exceedingly clean and willing to help in many American cities and towns, especially in the Midwest (including Canada). They drink a lot of milk on their corn cereal in the morning and by the glass before going to bed. There is a freshness, an "I am here, can I help you?" attitude that one doesn't encounter on other continents.

A friend of mine from Norway raised sons in the United States, and one of them went back to Oslo. He had a very hard time because if someone needed help, crossing roads or something, he was always ready to lend a hand. The Norwegians looked at him as an odd fellow. He had to put away this American impulse to be helpful and become a bit coldhearted in order to fit in.

Furthermore, former Easterners from all over the Far East who have lived on the North American continent for several generations have the same look of freshness. Their slight, slender bodies have grown bigger like their American counterparts. Never mind that they look a bit Asian; they are Americans or Canadians. The same is true for those of other racial backgrounds; they become bigger, taller, and friendlier just by living on the American continent. Besides the food, the forces coming to this part of the world are such that they produce bigger, stronger human beings, plants, and animals.

As mentioned previously, a vegetarian diet will provide more energy because the digestive system has to work harder to digest the food, as opposed to a meat diet in which there is less strain. It has been discovered among anthropologists that certain tribes that have a more vegetarian diet are more peaceful, as opposed to meat eaters who are more warrior-like. Warring people such as the Germanic tribes consumed meat, which gave them courage to fight. Other tribes residing in other parts of the Earth, such as in Africa where fruits, nuts, and a vegetarian diet led to a more artistic society, developed a more gentle character. Some of these people created beautiful arts, painting, and sculpture. We look at

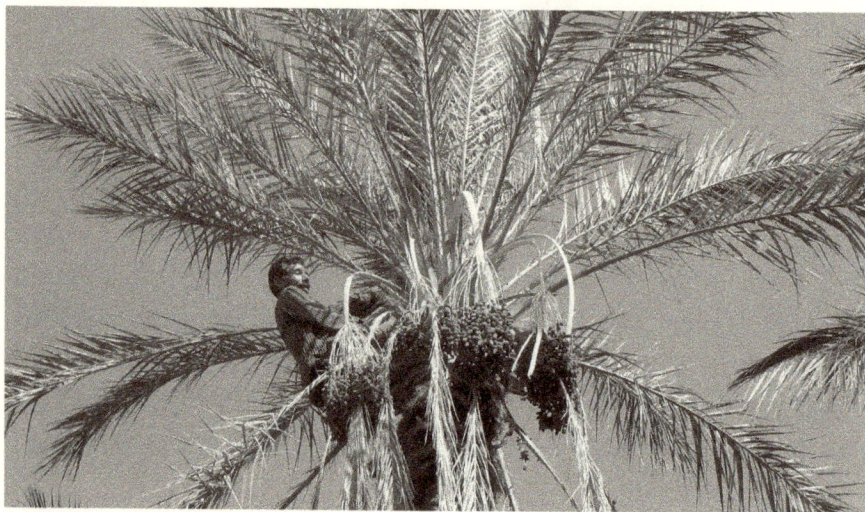

Time to harvest fresh dates; Tozeur, southern Tunisia,
an oasis in the Sahara and a world producer of dates

Americans and their tendencies in the diet—more meat eating with occasional pockets of vegetarianism such as in California, Vermont, or other hidden corners where young people are adopting a more gentle lifestyle—and we can foresee that we are preparing a future warrior society.

We know that many young men and women are being sent around the world to fight for "freedom" and "democracy." Is it beneficial to humankind to bring up fighters who shed blood to bring freedom? Is it right to take advantage in this way of our youth and their intrinsic willingness to help, their openness, and perhaps even their naivety? Does the Western diet prepare young people to be nothing but fighters, warriors?

Where are the artists? The musicians? The gentle poets? "Meat enchains one to Earth." But why is this?

Milk production depends far more on the animal's vital forces than it does on drives and instincts. We said...that animal protein is the most easily digested food because it is a substance lifted above the plant stage, and to a high level of organization by the digestive work animals have done on it, requiring little further digestive effort on the part of the human consumer.

But we must consider the following facts. Plants lift lifeless minerals to their own life level. When they eat plants, human beings have to assume the work of reorganization at the point where the plants leave off and carry it to a point two stages higher, through the animal to the human level. Though animals, too, reorganize the plants they eat, they do so in a way very different from human beings. Animal protein thus represents a real burden on the human body. The more developed and creative a person is, the more oppressive this load seems. Meat weighs us down with earthly heaviness and stirs up instinctive will forces that express themselves as passion and emotion. It is thus a food that chains us to the Earth. As Steiner said, it has the effect of making us feel quite satisfied to lose heaven if we gain the earth thereby.[12]

Human beings are extraordinarily complicated creatures. When people begin to live as vegetarians, there are many things to be considered. With everything that we consume—animal, plant, and mineral—we take in the spiritual forces that formed it. If, for example, we eat beef, the forces are drawn into us that worked on that being back when the animal fell from that series of advancing beings. Animals are beings who descended before their time, in which the forces hardened, the forces at work on them at the time of their turning aside [from the evolutionary process]. Animals have remained at the stage of evolution of that time. Thus, when the bull fell out, the forces worked in such a way that a small brain and a protruding snout were formed.... This is not to be understood in such a way that one becomes physically similar to a bull, acquiring a protruding snout and so forth; rather, one takes those forces into the astral body that then work to harden in this way. After death, when the astral body is freed, it assumes those forms. We can see this on the astral plane; this is the basis for the idea of "transmigration of souls."

However, human beings today need the hardening that comes from consuming flesh. Humankind was intentionally led to eating

---

12 Hauschka, *Nutrition*, pp. 54–55.

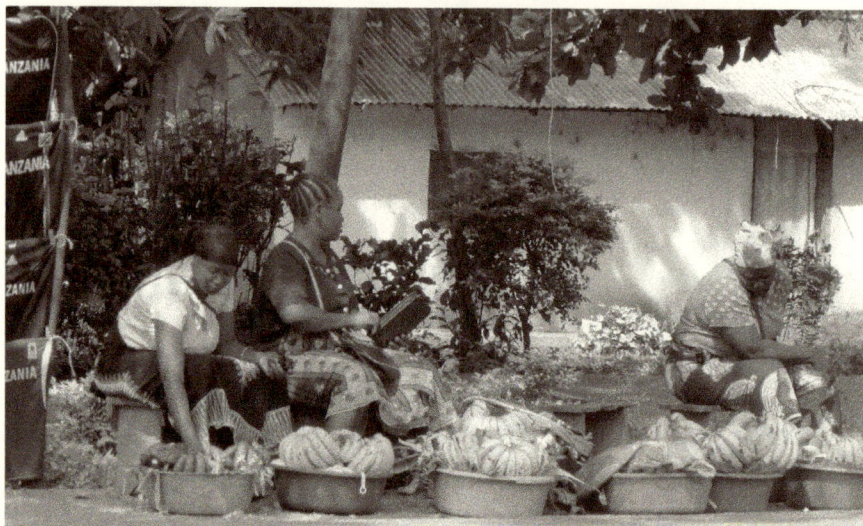

Northern Tanzania; local women selling vegetables and fruits near a main highway

animals at a certain time. In the beings that did not fall from the entire process—in whom the form, at the moment of falling out of the process, was not hardened—the forms remained softer so that other forces could continue to work on them and develop them to higher stages. If human beings had not eaten animals they would have remained soft; they would have assumed grotesque forms instead of the present-day human countenance. Now, if people today live as vegetarians then they lose this hardening influence, this inner solidity; and if they do not have a healthy body through heredity, if they are not, as we say, robust, they can easily lose their inner stability.[13]

Here we have both aspects of adopting the vegetarian diet: its positive aspects of producing more energy if one has the strength to digest the food and keep firmly grounded without the meat, and the negative aspects that arise if one is not strong enough to maintain stability without the grounding effect of meat and milk. There is a

---

13   Steiner, *Esoteric Lessons 1904-1909*, pp. 397–398.

fine line here. Heredity sometimes makes the wisest choice: meat for one, no meat for the other. We will discuss this from various viewpoints throughout the book.

> Humankind, although appearing more animal-like to begin with, was highly civilized.
>
> Now perhaps you will ask: But were those original animal-like people the descendants of apes or of other animals? That is a natural question. You look at the apes as they are today and think we are descended from those apes. But when human beings had their animal form, there were no such animals as today's apes. Human beings have therefore not descended from the apes. On the contrary, apes are beings who regressed.
>
> Going back further in Earth's evolution, we find human beings...developing from a soft element—not from our present animals. Human beings could never evolve from the apes of today. On the other hand it would easily be possible, if conditions on Earth today continued—conditions in which everything is based on violence and power, and wisdom counts for nothing—well, it could indeed happen that those who want to base everything on power would gradually assume animal-like bodies again, and that two races would then appear. One race would be those who stand for peace, the spirit, and wisdom, while the other would be those who revert to an animal form. It might indeed be said that those who care nothing today for the progress of humankind, nor spiritual realities, may be running the risk of degenerating into an ape-type species.[14]

It is because of these powerful statements that I write this little book on nutrition. As you will see, there is much more at stake than just food.

If the Western world continues to look at food as simply chemical ingredients to count, measure, and weigh, which is a materialist attitude, we will fall into utter disaster. We have already entered an

---

14   Steiner, *From Sunspots to Strawberries...*, pp. 119–120.

atmosphere of violence, intolerance, and hate among people; we see the effect every day in the news.

> A spiritual or a materialistic mental attitude is certainly not without importance for the next incarnation. Those who have some knowledge of the higher worlds—we need only believe in their existence—will have in their next life well-centered physical bodies and tranquil nervous systems—bodies that they have well in control, including even the nerves. On the other hand, those who believe in nothing but what they find in the sensory world communicate this kind of thinking to their physical bodies, and in their next incarnation will have bodies prone to nervous disorders—frail, fidgety bodies that have no steadfast center of volition. Materialists disintegrate into many separate fragments; the spirit binds together because spirit is unity.
>
> In individuals, this tendency appears in the next incarnation, but it also continues through the generations, so that the children and grandchildren of materialistic fathers and mothers have to pay for this through a poorly constituted nervous system and nervous disorders. An era of nervousness such as ours is the result of the materialistic attitude of the last [nineteenth] century. To counteract this, the great teachers of humanity have recognized the necessity of allowing the inflow of spiritual ways of thinking.[15]
>
> If the stream of spirituality is not powerful enough to influence the lazy and easy-going people as well, then nervous disorders, the karmic consequence, will gain greater and greater hold over humanity; and just as in the Middle Ages there were epidemics of leprosy, so, in future, materialistic thinking will give rise to grave nervous diseases—epidemics of insanity will beset whole nations.[16]

I leave the reader to fill in the blanks and observe what is happening now on the world stage. Just read the papers.

---

15 Steiner, *Rosicrucian Wisdom*, p. 66.

16 Ibid., p. 67.

What is the difference between being softly rooted to the earth through the use of milk products and being chained to the earth through meat intake? We lose sight of the "heavenly."

Another American favorite is jam and peanut butter sandwiches. My family never had this favorite American food. Our French palate was more demanding, and we just could not swallow this odd mixture. My father's homemade *pâté, boeuf bourguignon,* and *coq au vin* were more to our taste. I never served my children peanut butter, but replaced it with almond or hazelnut butter which we used on top of pancakes. Let us look at this plant, the peanut, and what it brings to our bodies.

The peanut plant originated in Central America. It is important in oil production, which is high in fat (50 percent) and high in protein (26 percent). It is used in the food industry worldwide, in the making of chocolate, margarine, table oil, animal feed, and fertilizer. It is now grown in Asia, Africa, Spain, and the United States. Its home is in the warmer climate where it produces more oil under the influence of the warm Sun.

After a relatively short germination period, the peanut sprout develops, with its typical leaf structure. Soon, the so-called sleep movement can be observed with the coming of darkness. It then does not strive upward toward the light, in typical fashion, but rather spreads out in bushy form. The developing tap root has numerous secondary roots with bacterial nodes. The flower formation takes place in the leaf axils and exhibits the well-known butterfly form with a golden-yellow flower.... Then the fruit nodes...then comes an unexpected, dramatic development. During the night, the flower bud develops an impressive longitudinal growth. In the early morning, the flower develops; but in the same morning, the flower begins to wilt, after having undergone a self-pollination during the brief blossoming. Then a stem-like form comes out of the flower and grows, pushing the remains of the flower with it. This is the so called fruit bearer. However, this growth does not proceed upward. On the contrary, the fruit bearer tends to increase downward, toward the Earth, until it finally reaches the ground. Then the tip bores into the earth and grows a few more centimeters under the earth. Only then does the ovule expand, and it begins to grow horizontally under the Earth's surface. The fruit-bearer now behaves like a root. It takes its nutrients from the earth—both water and substances. Calcium seems to play a large role here. As the bearer of animal desires...it has a significant influence on the ripening of the fruit underground. However, only one-fourth of the ovules sunk into the ground reach maturity.

We thus see this plant brings three properties to expression. First, it has a weak relation to light, which we see in its lack of directed horizontal growth—a property which it shares with many other legumes (beans, peas, etc.). Second, it is obviously overpowered by the gravitational forces of the Earth, in that it actively penetrates into the earth with its fruit-bearer. Third, once the fruits come into the earth, they ultimately behave like roots—they deny the cosmic, solar, nature and turn to earthly forces. In the darkness of the earth, the Moon forces are active, as we see in the formation of mushrooms. This relationship to the fungus world is clearly shown in the susceptibility of peanuts to fungi in the soil.[17]

The gesture of this plant is not a friendly one, and it should be avoided in the diet. We will discuss this further when we bring the soybean plant, mushrooms, algae, and more chemistry into the picture.

We can see that the American diet of meat, potatoes, peanut butter, corn, salty foods, and milk is concentrated in foods all containing forces that chain humans to the Earth. Milk is the only substance which creates a balance, offering the body gentle cosmic forces, or heavenly forces. When we look at the gesture of the sunflower with its face toward the Sun, the sunflower oil, in contrast to the peanut oil, offers different forces which are obvious. One is sunny; the other is dark, under the earth like potatoes. We see in this diet, therefore, an overabundance of dark forces chaining people to the Earth as

---

17   Schmidt, *The Essentials of Nutrition*, pp. 133–134.

opposed to the more "heavenly" forces of the Eastern diet with its emphasis on rice that is full of light-air properties that keep our contact with the cosmos and don't really penetrate the earth.

With this type of diet, is it not possible that the drug revolution and its craving to escape one's body is actually the search for a more balanced diet. When the body is chained to the Earth, then it desperately wants to be out. But it comes in a negative form, exiting the body through the strength of very poisonous plants like the coca plant, tobacco/nicotine, cocaine, derivatives of marijuana, or the plant itself with its cosmic properties. These or synthetic drugs represent a search for the light in darkness form.

Steiner mentions in his lectures that humankind is going to go through an initiation, a transformation, whether we like it or not. Of course it is better to be prepared and go through transformation on our own and not be forced to do so by external circumstances. Such things as natural disasters and unwelcome addictions bring these changes.

Here, in this diet, something is missing, and the body's cravings turn to the darkness, while pursuing the light. It is time for North Americans to change their diet and bring in a more balanced knowledgeable attitude toward nutrition. Later we will see how certain countries have achieved this.

Don't presume that because I have spoken of darkness and of a cloud I mean the clouds you see in an overcast sky or the darkness of your house when your candles fail. If so, you could with a little imagination picture the summer skies breaking through the clouds or a clear light brightening the dark winter. But this isn't what I mean at all, so forget this sort of nonsense. When I speak of darkness, I mean the absence of knowledge. If you are unable to understand something or if you have forgotten it, are you not in the dark in regard to that thing? You cannot see it with your mind's eye. Well, in the same way, I have not said "cloud," but *cloud of unknowing*. For it is darkness of unknowing that lies between you and your God.[18]

North Africa and the Sahara Desert

Now we travel from the North American continent, the land of plenty (not necessarily the land of nutritious food, but perhaps empty food and wasting food) to the desert lands. This part of the world, like the Far East and the West, is no longer accepting of dictators, kings, selfish leaders, despots, rulers, and patriarchs because the Western ways have invaded their land, and they are demanding freedom and just treatment of human beings. They are doing it their way, which is different from the West and the East.

This past fall I was fortunate enough to spend some time traveling in Morocco through the Atlas Mountains, through Tunisia, and the great Sahara Desert of the south. I wanted to see the land of my birth and the land where the "spark for freedom" ignited and spread like wildfire throughout the Middle Eastern world. I was there also to prepare for another book journey (*Beyond the Blood*).

In the capital Tunis the great main avenue was still full of barbed wire and tanks, and police cars carrying military or police forces were everywhere, while the people were enjoying themselves, sitting by the hundreds in French-style cafés and restaurants. Young men, families, couples, women covered and uncovered, girlfriends, intellectuals, and teachers were sipping tea and coffee, eating ice cream, smoking and laughing, and enjoying the evening or afternoon as if nothing mattered in the world. Tank drivers looked on, bored.

I spent two weeks in the desert by joining a French adventure group crossing the Sahara Desert on camels and on foot, living like the people of the old caravans did. We slept in nomadic tents, which we helped put up and take down ourselves, and some of the

---

18 Anonymous, *The Cloud of Unknowing*, p. 44.

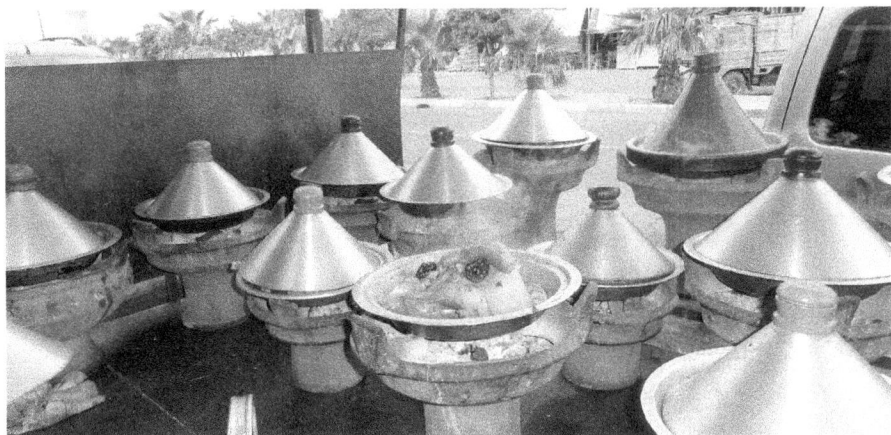

*Famous Berber tajines; fresh vegetables cooked in earthen pots on coals;
central Morocco near a beautiful oasis and waterfall with wild monkeys*

members of our party slept under the stars as the camel herders do, and we ate what they eat in the desert, which is not much of anything. There were eleven travelers, nine camels, one tourist guide, and five camel drivers who were also guides and cooks. It was a real desert experience in that respect. We had paid enough for food, but the local organizers kept the money and fed us very little, which in a way was a learning experience for all of us. The camel herders did not seem to mind. That was their diet.

Every morning one of the camel herders, the baker, would prepare homemade bread in a large bowl, putting in flour with water and working on it for a while. This cooking began in the cool desert temperature under the stars while we were still sleeping. He had started a large fire first with the small pieces of wood and dead brush that we had gathered the previous evening, and made sure there were plenty of coals. Then he formed the dough into a huge flat pancake, which he dropped on the burning hot coals. Then he covered the bread with hot sand, coal, and ash and let it cook for a half an hour. Then as we watched, he cleaned out the sand, coal, and ashes from the bread and it was done, a beautiful hot loaf. That was our breakfast, along with jam and some butter and tea made from some kind of leaves not resembling tea I was familiar with. We ate this morning and evening, and for lunch we had tomato salad with bread leftover from breakfast and some water. Supper was a broth with a couple of potatoes. There was no meat, fruits, or dessert. That is what we ate for the ten days. Sometimes for a treat we had two tablespoons of pomegranate seeds.

The camel handlers worked when eating only that diet. Their skin was dark like weathered leather and their faces had deep wrinkles. They were thin and wiry, with not one bit of fat on their strong bodies. Shaped by the Sun, the wind, sand, and working with their gentle beasts, they ate little and walked much through the dunes. They had walked four days to the spot where we met them and at the end had to walk to their village on the edge of the great Sahara Desert. It was a privilege to be with such people who were wise from living under the stars. They all had children, wives, and a few animals to make a living. Their lives were hard, but they were healthy and thankful to God for what they had. They did not consume, as Westerners do, most of the planet's raw materials. The little bit of desert brush that we collected at night was sufficient to make bread and provide a bit of warmth in the evening. We listened to their simple instruments accompanied by songs, primitive powerful singing, and we danced under the stars around the fire at night like they did thousands of years ago. Not much seemed to have changed. If you went straight from the Sahara, in either direction, right across the Middle East to Persia and across Algeria, into Morocco to the Atlantic Ocean, there would be nothing for thousands of miles but desert land and its people who live on very little but are grateful.

As I sat on the camel, soothed by the rhythm of its gait day after day, I listened to the beautiful voices of the camel herders as they talked to each other in their deep guttural language while walking with a stick over their shoulder alongside their beast. The head camel driver, who was in his early seventies and looked wiser than the rest, would stop the caravan around 3:00 and perform his prayers, looking toward Mecca, reciting the ancient words which are repeated millions of times throughout the Moslem world and sent as a fervent cloud into the universe:

> The first chapter of the Qur'an is the *surat al fatihah*, "chapter of the opening," which consists of seven verses (*ayat*). It is without doubt the most often recited chapter of the Qur'an, because it constitutes the heart of the daily canonical prayers and contains, in a synoptic fashion, the message of the whole of the Qur'an:
>
>> In the name of Allah, the infinitely Good,
>> the all-merciful
>> Praise be to God, the Lord of the worlds,
>> The infinitely Good, the all-merciful,
>> Master of the day of judgment.
>> Thee we worship, and in Thee we seek help.
>> Guide us upon the straight path,
>> the path of those on whom Thy grace is,
>> not those of whom Thy anger is,
>> nor those who are astray.[19]

Listening to these incantations, I became a herder myself and grew to love this wild expanse of quiet desert where only little creatures nothing seems to live except. I was reminded of the 40 days in the desert where the desert fathers lived to be closer to God. These people were close to God; they did not speak much and they could read minds from living in solitude during their long treks across the great dunes. They did not need to speak. It must have been a wonderful emptying, with the ever-present stars above.

> There are people...who never look up to the stars during their whole life—who do not know the location of Leo, Aries, or Taurus; they have no interest in any of this. Such people are born, in their next life on Earth, with a body that is somehow limp and flabby. Or if, through the vigor of their parents, they receive a model that

---

19 Nasr, *Islam: Religion, History, and Civilization*, pp. 40–41.

carries them over this, they become limp, lacking energy and vigor, through the body that they then build for themselves.[20]

Camel drivers and sheep herders sleep under the stars; their bodies are lean and compact. They are energetic and, as we see their faces that have acquired ancient wisdom, we are touched by their beauty. These words of Rudolf Steiner remind me of what I feel from their ancient faces, which have gazed at the desert skies strewn with stars year after year.

> Picture it quite graphically. You are caressed by someone who loves you. You feel the caress, but it would be childish to associate it in any way with physical matter. The caress does not matter at all; it is a process, and you experience it inwardly in your *soul*. Thus it is when we look out into etheric spheres. The gods, in their love, caress the world. But their caress lasts long, because the life of the gods spans immense reaches of time. In truth, the stars are the expression of love in the cosmic ether; there is nothing physical about them. From the cosmic aspect, to see a star means to feel a caress that has been prompted by love. To gaze at the stars is to become aware of the love coming from the divine-spiritual beings. What we must come to realize is that the stars are only the signs and tokens of the presence of the gods in the universe.[21]

We arrived in the oasis, which we could see from miles away, at the end of the trek. And there it was, date palm trees with great succulent fruits, richer than anything on Earth, the dates' sweetness like a warm spring coming from deep within the Earth. The dates grew for miles in an area which is desert, miles of sand dunes, and all of a sudden we saw an explosion of greenery. One cannot find a greater contrast.

The diet of the area is centered on the meat of lamb, sheep, and goats that graze on brush and even climb into the lower trees. It is

---

20 Steiner, *Karmic Relationships*, vol. 1, p. 86.
21 Ibid., vol. 7, p. 29.

a sign of wealth to own such herds, and the herders take pride in their animals.

I was lucky to be in Tunisia this last fall to celebrate the festival of the sheep. Sheep were being slaughtered by the thousands from one side of the North African continent to the next for one week. The poor as well as the rich will slaughter their sheep and use every single bit of the animal's meat. Nothing is wasted. As I traveled throughout the country on public transport I saw small trucks full of sheep skins on their way to being delivered to tanneries for the leather trade. All is used, put away in freezers, or hung in the sunlight to dry. After the trek we visited a small family compound where the people lived in caves, and I saw how they used everything and realized how wasteful we are back in the West. These people of the desert know what it is to live beyond frugality. They deserve to win a sustainability prize.

This celebration is an occasion for families to go back to their villages, visit relatives, and celebrate in common their thankfulness for life, for the elders, for their communal life, and for their faith as Moslems. Everyone was traveling. Young women studying in Tunis returned home in the far south near Libya. They all crisscross the country to be home for the festival. The whole town where I was staying at the beginning of the festival on the island of Djerba (bordering Libya) was empty. No one was working; restaurants were closed. It was the Christmastime of the Middle East. Children had received their presents and everyone was busy eating and celebrating.

The staple of the Middle East is couscous, made from wheat and served with lamb, chicken, or beef broth, cooked with chickpeas, carrots, cabbage, turnips, sometimes potatoes, and other root vegetables. I love this simple dish and have cooked it for my family quite often. It is a very satisfying meal in which you can omit the meat, which is done when families do not have meat available. Warm flatbread is also served when couscous is not, and then one uses the bread as a fork or spoon and dips it into the large communal dish as I noticed the camel herders did when they ate among themselves.

All the remote villages from the Atlas Mountains of Morocco, to the coastal towns of Algeria, to Tunisian hamlets near the Sahara Desert, to the desert of Mt. Sinai, or the city of Jerusalem—all across the Middle East there are small bakeries fueled by wood fire or gas furnace. Everyone has fresh bread available at a nominal cost. In my small town in Wisconsin we were not even able to sustain one bakery because people in the West have lost touch with the real meaning of bread. Wonder Bread in the United States is a classic example of fluff, emptiness, and poisonous food.

These people know that bread is the most important ingredient in one's diet, and they want it fresh. If the government does not sponsor inexpensive wheat flour for bread, the people go to the streets and demand it. But now they are buying flour from the West, which is contaminated by incorrect agricultural practices, so their health will deteriorate unless they start growing their own. The same is true for the white rice of the Far East, which is causing colon ulcers and other physical problems.

Because these people have a balanced diet (in the big cities, youth is changing) they are relatively healthy. They also have a *hammam*, a communal bath, that is usually heated by a large wood-burning furnace, or a gas or diesel furnace which runs all day. This is true in all the small towns where not everyone has a shower. The *hammam* is full on Wednesday, in preparation for Friday's prayer, and Thursday evening is the couple's night for celebration. The men and women (separately—women in the daytime, men in the evening) go to the *hammam* for a small fee. There one can get scrubbed and massaged by local women or men, and women spend hours being refreshed by the clean water. It is extremely healthy for the body to get rid of the dead layer of skin. The skin can breathe again and then it can absorb the outside forces, substances which nourish the body. When traveling alone in the man's world of the Middle East it is one of my favorite places to go to meet and spend time with women. The men always comment that the women spend too much time in the *hammam*, and in conversation I often said, "But you men spend time in the café," and they agree. *Hammam* for women, cafés for men, except in larger cities and wealthier towns where men and women both hang out in cafés.

There is nothing like a sweet store in the Middle East, which is where the art of sugar really came into being (more about sugar later) after coming from India. There are lots and lots of sweets made from almonds, pistachios, walnuts, butter, honey, dates; the array is simply astonishing. And it is extremely rich and full of ingredients that make for strong hearts: fruits and sesame, sunflower, and other seeds. These people have not lost the art of making sweets. Some areas do not have proper dental hygiene and people lose their teeth because of the large amount of sugar they drink with mint tea. But thanks to advertising and the younger generation that likes beautiful white teeth, there is an awakening about this issue.

From this diet we can see that many generations of Middle Easterners will be healthy, unlike the unhealthy trends of the North American diet and its epidemics of heart disease, cancer, nervous disorders, infertility, and other illnesses.

Now let us reflect a bit on sheep, which are the animals seen most frequently in large herds throughout these lands.

Sheep produce the most beautiful fur, or wool.... The sheep forms its hair by the powers of the inner light.... With sheep, the important thing is not the milk, nor is it the fat; it is the wool. If we ask about the sheep's special sense, I would have to tell you it is the sense of sight; it is in the eyes. It may not seem that a sheep is very much directed by its eyes, but if we consider the wild forms of sheep and goats, especially those that climb mountains, we can see that their skill depends on mastery of space. Although our modern domestic sheep have gradually lost this ability, we must still realize the significance of this sense of sight streaming in. The eyes, as they collect all the four lower senses, develop a special organ—the heart. Observe the sheep. See how light collects the four lower senses through the eyes, forms the heart, and builds, as it were, a monument here where all this manifest in the sheep—the tremendous horns that develop in all sheep in one form or another. The result, dear friends, is the fleece, or wool. The sheep's brain formation is no longer an organ. The brain formation in sheep is the whole of the fleece. What does the saga of the argonauts whereby Jason went in search of the golden or holy fleece mean? Jason was looking for what was once cosmic wisdom. If, for instance, we look at the head of Zeus as it was formed in old Greek times, we will see that Zeus also is surrounded by a fleece—the powers of cosmic wisdom.[22]

As I traveled thousands of miles across desert and mountain landscapes throughout the Middle East, I loved watching the shepherds with their large herds of docile, quiet sheep, munching dried grass, knowing they give much to us, such as food, milk, wool for weaving beautiful artistic creations such as carpets and clothes, and large horns that may become musical instruments. Sheep are part of the scarce landscape and the psyche of this part of the Earth. I would say it is the heart of this land. Therefore, the festival of the sheep is a very important event in the Middle East. Similar to Christmas in the West, it is their festival of the inner light, and the entire Moslem world participates and looks forward to this joyous event. "You may understand now why people have always connected the lamb with the highest vision of the Christ. It is the inner light that builds the wool."[23]

This is a beautiful meditation, and we can learn much about that part of the world from it. The sheep comes under the sign of the "Lion" in the zodiac, and the wool reminds us of the lion's mane.

Mohammed is called *heart*.

---

22 König, *Earth and Man*, pp. 29, 49–50.

23 Ibid., p. 29.

Because the land does not have the ability to grow black tea as do countries such as Iran and India, mint tea is a favorite drink in North Africa. It is offered and served in a special way by holding the teapot up in the air and pouring the clear greenish-yellowish boiling liquid into the glass without burning anyone. Mint tea, very sweet and boiling hot, is refreshing and is served everywhere in Morocco. The mint plant thrives in any of the wet embankments where the farmers have built irrigation ditches throughout the oasis. The Moroccans consume this beverage by the gallon. In the market one sees wheelbarrows or donkeys' backs loaded with the plant for sale. It is served after a couscous meal or during the day with sweets, or for breakfast with flat bread. In the *souks,* one is often offered mint tea and a welcome chat, which I never refuse. Mint belongs to the *Labiatae* family of plants.

> One gets the clearest impression of *Labiatae* by tasting and smelling them. They all have a warming fragrance and flavor.... It's as though the whole plant had been dipped in aromatic fire forces from root to blossom.... Plants of this family are not the sort to whip up and stimulate. Each possesses in its individual aroma the power to calm and harmonize. They lighten heaviness, drive away chills, and relieve monotony, all effects that aid the metabolic forces.
>
> Etheric oils are carriers of these harmonizing elements that permeate *Labiatae,* and they in turn owe this capacity to hydrogen... "fire substance."...
>
> Etheric oils are the richest in hydrogen of all plant substances. They lift toward the wide reaches of the cosmos as though on wings of warmth, raising the plant with them as they do so....
>
> One single gesture is common to all *Labiatae*—giving themselves out, going up in scent or aroma. The comparable trait in human beings is digestion as it takes place on the other side of the intestinal wall. Thus, the *Labiatae* aid assimilation and transubstantiation processes in the blood; they accompany food substances as these are broken down from their initial "appearance," or material state, into one where they become pure force or being.

Labiatae, then, support the "I" in its task of building up uniform human protein.

The various mints, melissa, marjoram, thyme, and salvia, as well as rosemary and summer savory, thoroughly warm the digestive tract. They are particularly effective in supporting the heart.[24]

Moroccans do not complain of liver disorders as do their neighbors the French; mint tea takes care of their digestion, a quality of this marvelous aromatic plant that everyone should include in their diet. It is much healthier than a soda and should *never* be served along with "modern" beverages, which are simply sweetened water.

SPAIN

From North Africa, we cross the Straits of Gibraltar and arrive in Spain, where I had the privilege to walk again this last spring from Seville to Santiago de Compostela, from south to north. The paths go near many private haciendas, olive groves, mountains, arid terrain, some wetlands, lovely white villages sitting on hills, fortresses from the Middle Ages, and Moslem-influenced architecture. As I walked through the forests, I came across herds of pigs, smaller brown pigs living freely in large enclosed forested areas foraging for food and living a healthy life until it is time for butchering. These animals are famous worldwide, because they do not have much fat and so are healthier as meat. As I stopped for a quick meal, I had to eat the meat because there was simply nothing else available except eggs and potato *frittata.* I therefore ate a lot of ham prosciutto cheese sandwiches in the many cafés on the way, where I was usually the only woman among workmen taking a break for lunch. Walking through the private land which the path accessed, I was a little apprehensive about the

---

24 Hauschka, *Nutrition,* pp. 102–103.

herds of semi-feral pigs that came running to see what was going on. I ran behind some gates for safety, then turned around and looked at the pigs staring at me from beneath lovely long eyelashes. They then continued on with their business of feeding. I walked through hundreds of miles with these companions scattered here and there. Sometimes I noticed very large structures and a funny smell. The pigs living on these industrial farms were not as fortunate as their brothers and sisters in the forests who freely roamed in thyme, rosemary, and lavender scented meadows. The pig belongs to these native lands, as do the wild boars, which are seen throughout Europe. Boars are more dangerous, but in all my walks I have never encountered them. I have seen their tracks but not the animals themselves.

Spain, France, Italy, and Germany consume a lot of pork and have created a successful industry from this animal. Pig has been companions to human beings for thousands of years. The pork industry in the United States is also extremely well developed, but I find that Spain is at the top of the list. In all the little villages, the meat shops had hundreds of cured hams hanging from the ceilings, and much of their meat is shipped worldwide.

> The pig is a naked animal. Although it certainly has bristles, the actual domestic pig is naked, even rosy. No skin color in any animal is so similar to the human skin as that of the pig.... There is something that is utterly nonhuman—the tremendous snout, the round, open nose. As soon as we see this, we can connect the pig with all the animals that belong to the elephant group.... We can also see the strange form of the opening of the mouth....
>
> All this indicates that the foremost sensory organ of the pig is the nose—or, more accurately, the sense of smell. And what does this very special form of snout or the trunk of the elephant signify?
>
> Can you see how the pig can do everything with this very special part of its body? The elephant, the mammoth—they all had this extended trunk; in Atlantis the forests were jungles, and to find their way through the jungle it was necessary for them to

pave the way with their trunks, as well as to smell, touch, and experience through movement all that was around. The eyes did not matter, because they could not see. Everywhere was sprouting life, plants so thick that we can no longer imagine it. Through this, the elephant paved their ways. A reminder of this remains in the pig. If such a thing happens in an organism, however, other parts of it must at once begin to adjust, and so the pig develops a huge kidney.... If we open the embryo of a pig in the second month, we find almost the whole abdomen of the pig filled with a tremendous kidney—because everything is smell. Then perhaps we can begin to realize that this kidney is the brain of the pig.

The result of this is the deep layer of fat that covers the whole surface under the skin.[25]

The pig presents an especially amazing picture of heat and light. It really has no hair as other animals do; it has only bristles. Moreover, pigs cannot sweat, or perspire at all, except in a very small area around the snout....

Question: I can understand that the pig is intimately connected with humankind. Why, then, did the Jews find it to be an "unclean animal"?

It is an unclean animal as human food because it contains so many human elements that, when we eat it, the meat acts a little like alcohol; it wipes out the individual's identity, and the Jewish people had to prevent this. If you see people who eat pork, you will find that they are somewhat numbed in regard to "selfhood." Now don't think you must discard bacon; things are different today. However, the fire of alcohol and the fire of the pig are something very similar.[26]

So the pig gives us fat, and we transform that fat into warmth and light. In ancient times, we ourselves lit our rooms with the help of the oil of fatty substances.[27]

---

25 König, *Earth and Man*, pp. 45–46.

26 Ibid., p. 32.

27 Ibid., p. 51.

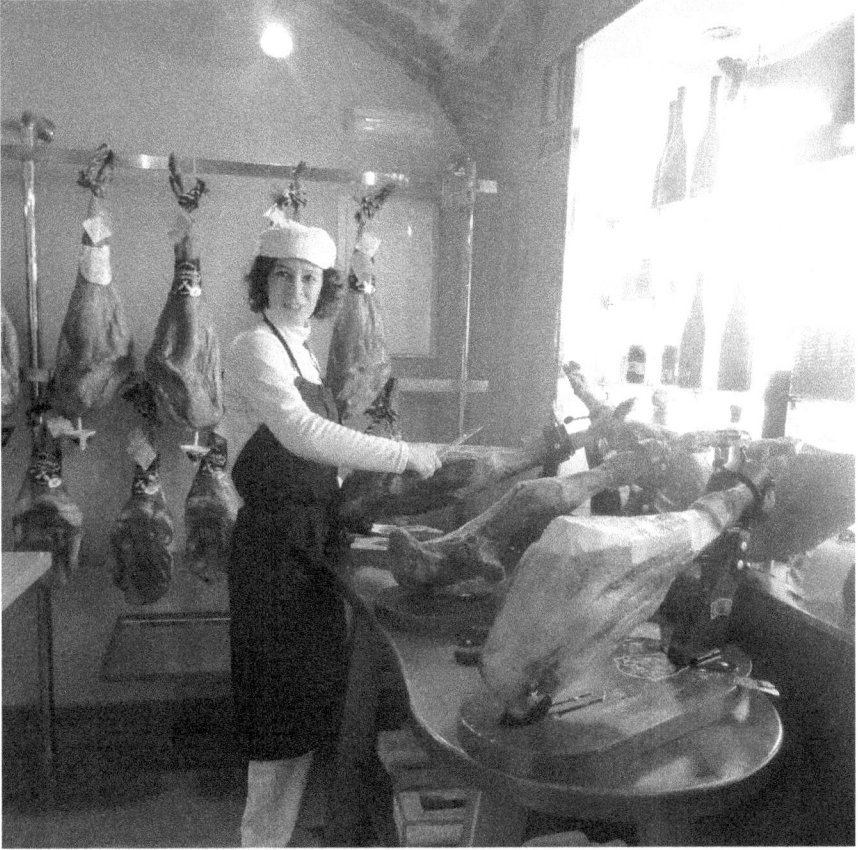

Southern central Spain; a dry meat shop selling non-fat ham

❦

The Spanish land is also the home of the sacred olive groves, which thrive in the Mediterranean climate. I walked through many olive groves admiring the trees' beautiful ancient shapes and enjoyed eating their most amazing nut-fruit. They gather sunlight and transform it into precious oil.[28]

---

28 For more about olive trees, see Valandro, *Letters from Florence.*

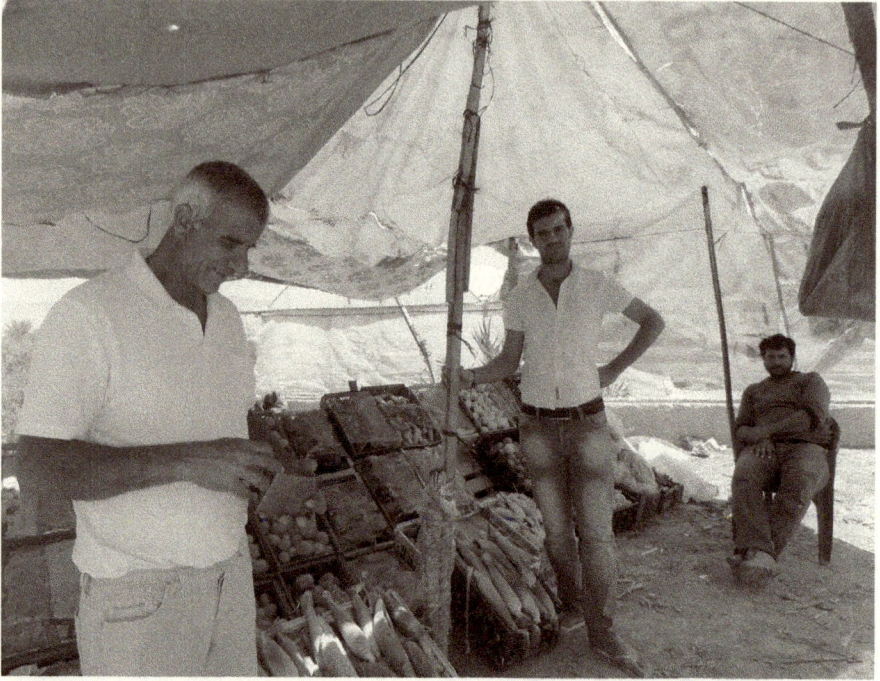

Palestine; on the road from Galilee to Jerusalem;
Palestinians selling produce on the roadside

The Earth is amazing. When it is not fertile enough, too dry and rocky, it makes up for it by providing something to balance it out, such as the rich olive tree. The desert where there seems to be nothing at all suddenly has an outburst of rich date palm trees. It seems the more desert-like, the richer the fruits to balance things out.

Among human beings we could say that if someone is missing something, that person has to work hard to compensate for it, thereby developing capacities that others do not have: a blind person will develop exquisite sensitivity to sounds; someone who does not speak very much will be able to read someone's feelings. Steiner mentions that people who want to develop certain abilities to use on behalf of humankind have to spend one extreme one-sided life as a handicapped person, and in their next life they will have special gifts. Communities that care for the disabled, such as those of the

Camphill Movement that follow the indications of Rudolf Steiner, have sprouted throughout the world, caring for their members in a loving, sustainable, and healthy way.

The olive tree was cultivated in the Near East thousands of years ago. From there it spread throughout the entire Mediterranean region. It appears to have grown originally in Abyssinia and Arabia, both as a tree and as a wild bush. At the beginning of Greek culture, around 700 BC, it covered the hills and coasts of the mainland and the islands with its ever-green wood.

The olive tree was highly regarded in the Jewish culture of the Old Testament, as well as in Greek culture. Olive oil was in general use for sacrifices in the temple, for food, for anointing the body, and for oil lamps. Early on, this tree was considered "holy" and dedicated to the goddess Athena. Her olive trees on the Acropolis were untouchable, as they were symbols of spiritual clarity and peace. In Olympia, victorious competitors were decorated with olive branches. A Greek myth relates that Jupiter preferred the gift of Minerva, who brought him an olive branch; its fruit was not only good to eat, but it also yields a miracle juice that seasons people's food, heals their wounds, gives strength to their bodies, and lights the night. According to biblical tradition, the "oil of mercy" comes from an olive tree growing from one of the seeds that Seth placed in the mouth of his father Adam....

The olive tree belongs to the Mediterranean region. It is protected from extreme cold from north of the Alps and borders the hot desert of the African coastal lands. The extremes are moderate, because of the multi-faced ocean surfaces that reflect the light and warmth, preparing the atmosphere of that region, from which ninety percent of all olives come. It is as if an image of both human poles—the cool brain and the fiery metabolism—reaches a mercurial balance in the Mediterranean region. The heart forces—the human center—seem to be incarnated in that olive tree landscape. The forces of Earth and Sun are reconciled, and earthly and cosmic warmth interpenetrate each other. Wilhelm Pelican describes the noble character of olive oil: "In it, hard knowledge is purified upward into the grace and peace of the Sun life. It gave strength to food, and provided a balancing mildness to the polarities of sharp, sour, and salty."[29]

This summarizes the magic of the olive-tree landscapes. I have experienced it throughout the Middle East, Palestine, Israel, Greece, Morocco, Tunisia, Algeria, France, and Italy. Christianity belongs to the olive-tree landscape perhaps for the very reasons mentioned. It balances between the hot and fiery and the cool. One feels comfortable walking for hours among the sacred groves of olive trees. In these olive groves, much healing can happen.

The Spanish earth also is home to rosemary plants which grow wild and healthy, as well at thyme and lavender, but unlike Italy and France, the Spaniards are not making much use of these beautiful heavenly scented plants.

The Spanish soil is certainly not conducive to cattle farming, except in the northern regions of Galicia, so the land gives its other gift, olive oil.[30] Fat from the oil replaces milk for consumption. Spaniards are small of stature and compact with beautiful complexions like the Italians. They have strong bodies and are full of life.

Their diet also includes lamb, hard cheese from sheep's milk, rice, fish, oranges, and other citrus fruits that grow in orchards throughout the south like their North African neighbors. With these natural gifts, the Spaniards enjoy a relatively healthy diet. They get their fat mostly from the olive tree and the pig, fish from the ocean, rice, potatoes, eggs, chicken, citrus fruits, peppers, walnuts, and almonds. They make the famous *paella*, a great saffron rice dish with fish, seafood, and meat.

In Madrid, where I stayed for a while, I was charmed by the very old ladies strolling two-by-two in the large squares that are filled with people at night. People are living to a ripe old age with this

---

29 Schmidt, *The Essentials of Nutrition*, pp. 139–140.
30 See Valandro, *Camino Walk*.

diet. Appropriately, with these very rich oils, we can discuss fat and its function in our diet.

What is the effect of fat in the diet? People have the capacity to produce their own fats. But we still need to have this process stimulated by fat that we consume in foods....

Fat is not a body-building material in the sense we have been told that protein is. Its role is to supply a foundation for the life processes taking place in various organs. Fat is deposited in the organism and then used as a source of warmth. All the functions of the human organs require embedding in a constant warmth, and fat plays an important part in producing it. A fat deficiency tends to make the organ functions torpid, with the result that the physical body becomes inflexible and brittle and the life body insufficiently active.

The important thing here is to find the right balance between fat consumption and waking activity. This balance is always highly individual, for our individual relationship to fat is a faithful mirror of the way one's "I" is active in the area of life.

The purely vegetative functions that build the body, then, depend on fat to do their work. Too much fat intake depresses the psycho-spiritual functions linked to metabolic processes in the body, and the life-sense takes on a phlegmatic coloring. It can be especially harmful to combine a diet high in fats with a great deal of sleep, for this encourages body-building at the expense of soul and spiritual activity and makes the fat imbalance permanent. Fat is then deposited all over the body, like so much ballast....

The liver is the organ most involved in taking care of fats. First it produces the gall that combines with the intestinal trypsin and breaks the fat down. Then, it is the organ that revitalizes human substance after it has had all the life taken out of it in the intestines. The liver reacts at once to an incorrect fat diet, while a sick liver cannot process fat at all.

The question of source is as important with fats as we found it to be in the case of proteins. Unhealthy deposits of non-invigorated fat are caused by the type of fat consumed.... During summer, plants flow out through their blossoms into universal space, and the universe responds with the oil that appears in the ripening seed. Animal fats, however, are the product of the animal's own organism and bear the imprint of its special nature. But these fats do not have such strong animalizing effects on the human consumer as does protein.[31]

Why are some people born with a tendency to being overweight and others thin? Here are some insights. Perhaps reading this book will provide a "slimming cure" for the next life.

Consider, for instance, those who ponder or think a great deal in one incarnation. In their next incarnation, they will be thin, delicately constructed individuals. Those who think little in one earthly life and instead live a life more concerned with grasping the outer world tend to accumulate a great deal of fat in the next life. This, too, has a significance for the future. Spiritual "slimming cures" are not easily managed in one earthly life; one must resort to physical cures, if indeed they are of any help. But for the next earthly life it is certainly possible to undergo a "slimming cure" if by pondering and thinking a great deal, especially if one thinks about something that requires effort.[32]

And now, a bit more about olive oil as a food.

Olive oil is digested almost entirely by the human body.... It stimulates the appetite, especially when used with salads.... It is especially suited to nourishing our middle region....

Mild, supple, enveloping, gentle, opening, and effective against cramps. Internally it is effective against infection, the bites and stings of poisonous animals, and catarrhal conditions in the organs of respiration and digestion. It is also helpful against constipation and hemorrhoids—that is, against blockages and stagnation. Externally, too, its effect is to loosen, sooth, and relieve tension

---

31 Hauschka, *Nutrition*, pp. 56-57.

32 Steiner, *Karmic Relationships*, vol. 2, p. 125.

in cases of burns. Olive-oil massages are also effective in cases of gout and rheumatism.[33]

Perhaps the land of the olive tree is the chosen home to many Germans, English, and other northerners who migrate to Spain in the winter by the thousands to enjoy the coast and the inland beauty because they instinctively feel its healing power.

Speaking of fat, while enjoying Madrid and its cafés, sweet shops, and restaurants, I saw many people eating a combination which at first I did not want to try. But after seeing so many enjoying this breakfast I decided I would. It is *chorizo y chocolate*, long sticks of fried dough served with hot chocolate that is so thick you really can't drink it, but have to eat it with a spoon. I tried this deeply satisfying, mellow, comfortable sweet and went to another planet. I would go back to Spain just to taste it again, it was so delicious. It was highly fattening, but I did not care since I had walked 660 miles and needed all the fat I could get. I felt I had earned it, so I enjoyed this meal, eating it slowly because it was too rich to gulp down, and wondered why on earth I had not ordered it before.

When a girlfriend of mine met me in Madrid to go to the Prado Museum, we delighted ourselves with this formidable breakfast while sitting outside in a café next to a beautiful old church. So let us say something about chocolate which is highly prized and widely consumed in Spain, as opposed to the lightly sweet mint tea of Morocco.

> There is a third, plainer partner of these more fashionable beverages [coffee and tea]: the common cocoa. It occupies a place somewhere between tea and coffee, for it, too, tends to loosen the life body from the physical. The ensuing reaction, however, is neither one of sympathetic backward glances, nor an antipathetic rejection, but more a feeling of its heaviness. In Europe, chocolate is the favored drink for family parties, weighted down as they

---

33 Schmidt, *Essentials of Nutrition*, p. 140.

are with tradition and conventionality. It conveys a sense of healthy, well-fed satisfaction, of being sheltered within a structure of inherited customs. We must admit, though, that chocolate is very nourishing; it contains 50 percent fat, as well as protein and carbohydrates, making it better for the whole human being than the other beverages are.[34]

After discussing the Far East, the Middle East, the American continent, and Spain, it becomes obvious that much influence comes through the land in which we are born: how the sunlight hits a particular place on Earth. In the far north or the middle of the planet, the temperate zones have a distinct influence on the plant life, the animals, and the psyche of nations. The foods people eat also shape character and personality. We are, however, becoming independent of these forces, especially if we have traveled from a young age and been removed from their influence. Nevertheless, the forces still remain part of our world. There are also other important factors.

In the future, people will know how little they actually receive—as far as the substance of the body is concerned—from the food they eat. People receive far more from the air and the light, from all that they absorb in a very finely divided state from air and light, and so on. When this is realized, people will more readily believe that people build up a second body quite independently of any inherited conditions. For they build it entirely from their world environment.[35]

Now there are people who, in this earthly life, take a keen interest in all that surrounds them in the visible cosmos. They observe the worlds of plants and animals;...they take an interest in the majestic picture of the starlit sky. They are awake, so to speak, with their soul, in the entire physical cosmos. The inner life of human beings who have this warm interest in the cosmos differ from the

---

34 Hauschka, *Nutrition*, p. 117.

35 Steiner, *Karmic Relationships*, vol. 1, p. 84.

inner life of those who pass by the world with a phlegmatically indifferent soul....

There are, for example, those who have been on a short journey. When you talk to them afterward, they will describe with infinite love a town where they have been, right down to the tiniest detail. Through such keen interest, you yourself will get a complete picture of what it was like in the town visited.

From this extreme we can go to the opposite. On one occasion, for instance, I met two elderly women; they had just traveled from Vienna to Pressburg, which is a beautiful city. I asked them what it was like in Pressburg and what had pleased them there. They could tell me nothing except that they had seen two pretty little dachshunds down by the riverside. Well, they did not have to go to Pressburg to see the dachshunds; they might as well have seen them in Vienna. They had seen nothing else at all.

Consider a man with little interest in the physical world around him. Perhaps he barely manages to be interested even in the things that directly concern his bodily life—whether, for instance, one can eat more or less well in one or another region. His interests do not go beyond this, and his soul remains poor. He does not imprint the world into himself. He carries very little in his inner life, and very little of what has radiated into him from the phenomena of the world will go with him through the gate of death into the spiritual realms. Thus he finds that working with the spiritual beings, with whom he is then together, is very difficult. Consequently, in the next life he will not bring strength and energy of soul with him to form his physical body, but only weakness—a kind of faintness of soul. This model works into him strongly enough. The conflict with the model finds expression in manifold illnesses of childhood; but the weakness persists. He forms, so to speak, a frail or sickly body, prone to all sorts of illnesses. Karmically, therefore, our interest of soul-and-spirit in one earthly life is transformed into our constitution of health in the next life. Those who are "bursting with health" certainly had a keen interest in the visible world in a former incarnation.[36]

---

36 Ibid., pp. 84–86.

During my Sahara Desert trip I noticed that the camels' caretakers were keenly interested in their environment; they observed the tiniest movement in the sky to detect coming sandstorms, they looked attentively at the minute traces of insects that traveled at night leaving lovely, graceful movement in the sands in tiny millimeters steps. We can say that these people living with such primordial ways will have very healthy bodies in their next incarnations. Throughout the Middle East one sees children busily playing in the dirt. These children are extremely sturdy and awake and their eyes are shiny with interest. Again, these little beings will have sturdy healthy bodies in their next life. By contrast, on the American continent one sees how bodies will deteriorate, not only due to consumption of the wrong food and unhealthy agricultural practices, but a loss of interest in the surroundings. Children and adults no longer look at their environment with interest; they go shopping, watch movies, listen to music, and adopt a completely passive lifestyle. As a result, in the future we can see that there will be weak bodies, and thereby illness on a massive scale. Mothers should not give in to their children's nagging for what is not healthy for them. In that department "less is more."

In the Middle East, children still run around and play and the streets are alive with their joyful voices, games, and fights. In the developed countries one finds that the children no longer play in the street. As a child, I spent hours playing in the dirt with the neighbors, inventing games or just running around. We designed entire towns in the dirt and put handfuls of soil into newspapers, which we pretended was food and sold. We rode bikes, pretending we were cowboys. We ran on the beach half-naked, looked for frogs, and swam among the rocks. We designed special pools with rocks in our bathtub (my mother had a fit), made our own skis to go down the soft hills, and skied through the pine forest on cardboard. We dressed ourselves for made-up weddings by borrowing vintage clothes from Grandma's attic, and learned how to knit clothes for our dolls. Once we made our own shoes out of wood for fun, because I felt I had to walk on wooden shoes (past karma?). We even jumped out of a second-story window in Morocco onto duvets we had placed there for landing. I can't say we were very interested in school learning.

Today, children have toys for everything and no longer make their own entertainment, and thereby their creativity does not develop. If children are given everything to play with, how are they ever going to invent anything? They won't. And when they are thoroughly saturated with everything, they will have lost interest in the world. That is the beginning of the death of the soul and, as quoted, the next life will be a sickly one. By buying and giving children everything, we kill their resourcefulness. It simply does not develop *because there is no need.* Using the same principle, when a muscle is not exercised it atrophies.

We can therefore say that looking at the world with real interest feeds us and develops some soul muscles that will become healthy forces in the future. When raising children it is of utmost importance to provide this healthy interest, especially if your child is not so inclined. As a parent one must do everything one can, to make children more responsive to their environment and not give in to their apathy, which comes from former lifetimes or from their character. This is where the task of the parent becomes extremely important. We are shaping little souls for the future, and we are fortunate enough to have Waldorf schools in the world that take care of children in a wholesome way; or at least they try.

I am thankful for the dedicated teachers at the Pine Hill Waldorf School in New Hampshire and the High Mowing High School, the Aurora Waldorf School in Buffalo, New York, and the Spring Prairie Waldorf School in Wisconsin for providing my children with a wonderful education.

FRANCE

Now I will travel on and speak about France, my mother country, even though I also think of North Africa in this way. France is the cheese center of the world, with more than 400 varieties, but this number is decreasing because industrial agriculture has reached many of its regions. I have walked throughout France, from Vezelay to the Pyrenees and from Le Puy to Spain (Valandro, *The Path of Power*, unpublished manuscript) and have noticed it myself, firsthand. It will not be long before French cheese becomes as tasteless as American or Dutch cheeses. The flavors of the goat, sheep, and cow cheeses come from the animals' healthy diet of different herbs, plants, and shrubs, and each particular area has its specialties: mountain cheese from the Swiss or Italian Alps, dry cheese from the southern areas, rich creamy cheese from the river valleys.

I once walked through the Massif Central, a former volcanic area, and there I saw hundreds of goats in long buildings, unable to leave the premises. It had a terrible stench. This was new agriculture designed for goat cheese imports. These factories are out of the way, and one can only access them through difficult country roads or walking paths. It's a shame, and the local farmers complain about them as well. Throughout Europe, France, Germany, and England more and more farmers are keeping their livestock inside where they have no access to fresh air or fresh food. These practices increase diseases and poison the milk and the cheese. Grazing animals need to be outside; they belong in the green meadows under the Sun, and the land needs their manure to enrich the soil.

> Just as we can say that the kidney is the brain in the pig, in the cow it is the stomach. What does it mean that the cow and sheep and many other animals ruminate?... We know that in the process of digestion we completely destroy the food we take in and make it our own. In animals, the process is slightly different, however,

because not all the food is completely destroyed; some of it is kept in its own form and function. Ruminating comes about to prevent the complete destruction of food. The cow tastes and lives entirely with its food; you need only to hear the munching of a cow or the noise of a cow ruminating to see how the animal connects itself with the food. We can say that the cow loves the food through the sense of taste to such an extent that it doesn't want to destroy it; instead, cows, antelope, sheep, and goats—all ruminants—unite with the earthly substance, and by uniting as deeply and intimately as possible with this substance they permeate the substance with their own spiritual forces.

Rudolf Steiner has told us that the cow carries spiritual forces in itself. From earliest times it was venerated as a holy animal, because human beings felt awe before the cosmic powers living unhindered and unspoiled in the cow's frame. Those forces do not live in the physical frame but in the astrality of the cow; the cow carries part of the zodiac in its being, and the starry powers, through the ruminating process, unite with earthly substance and permeate it. This is the destiny of cattle. Why do we have a brain? We have a brain so that light, sound, smell, taste, and all the forms of nature do not fall into our existence but are held off. It is similar for the stomach-brain of the cow; the cow's food is not completely digested but is permeated by the spiritual powers of the animals, just as our percepts are permeated by our own thoughts and thus—by means of the central nervous system of the brain— remain outside of us.[37]

We have seen that the pig has a developed sense of smell and makes fat, and the kidney is his brain—nitrogen. The sheep has wool, sense of sight, and the heart as a developed organ—hydrogen. The cow has the sense of taste, the brain is the stomach, and milk is its gift—oxygen. The horse is the last animal, and the lung—movement, carbon.

---

37 König, *Earth and Man*, pp. 48–49.

Here we become familiar with these substances: nitrogen, hydrogen, and oxygen:

Nitrogen	kidneys (uric acid), pig	smell—Aquarius
Hydrogen	heart, sheep	sight—Leo
Oxygen	stomach, cow	taste—Taurus
Carbon	lung, horse	warmth—Eagle-Scorpio

Meditating on these animals who are our companions is a powerful way to understand our life on Earth. They each sacrificed something for us, for our wellbeing, and without them we would not be humans.

France has always been known for its wonderful food, which still has traces of wisdom or initiation knowledge. The French love *potage* like the English love flower gardens. As I walked through France on various old pilgrimage paths, I always saw vegetable gardens, well-tended little plots with neat rows of lettuces, onions, leeks, radishes, carrots, beets, and cabbages, along with fruit trees, strawberries, and currant bushes like my grandmother's extensive gardens. In the early mornings, gardeners tended their plants with infinite care and love. It is part of the European landscape, not often seen on the American continent except in wealthier more awakened communities. Europeans still have a deep connection to their gardens and their food, and they like to shop at the market for fresh produce from local gardeners. They demand freshness and vegetables that taste like vegetables, not like the produce sold in the American supermarkets that has little flavor. In small villages the farmers display their products with artistic delight, and I spent many hours just walking, admiring the abundance and beauty of the food and the creativity and inventiveness of its producers: chestnuts stuffed with goose liver (too rich for me!), honey from different flowers, local breads, and sweets. On one occasion the market was so spectacular that I almost stayed for a few days, just to sample some of the beautifully displayed foods—a sight I never see on the American

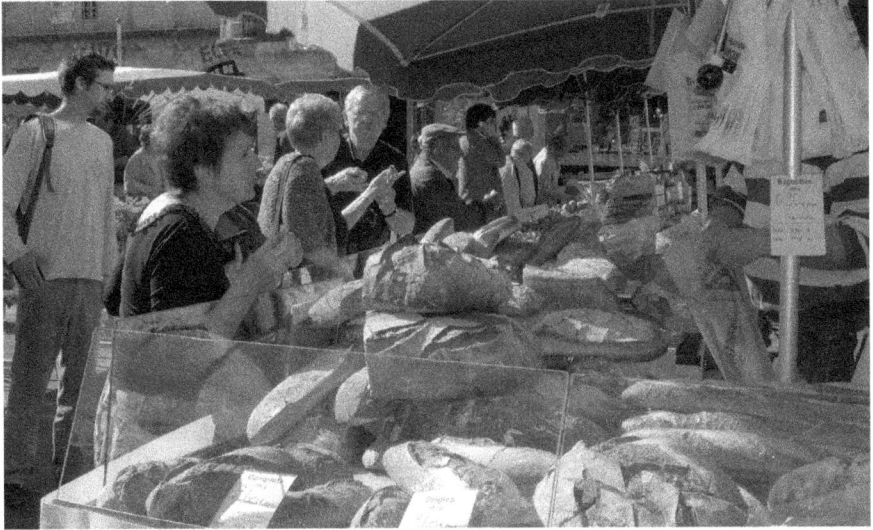

Perigord, central France, home of gastronomy; a city market with unimaginable delectable foods like stuffed chestnuts, dried fruits, and paté

continent. I spent the whole morning sitting in cafés watching the old people and the families shop and listening to the street musicians. I think the *perigord* (southwest) is the gastronomic center of France.

Some of my favorite recipes use leeks, a food beloved by the French. We have potato-leek soup served warm or cold, leek quiche, and leek salad which is made by steaming leeks, adding vinaigrette, and *voila!* Leeks are some of the richest plants containing iron, and if they are grown biodynamically, the iron content is much higher. If they are grown in conventional ways, they should not be eaten, because the iron in the plant forms a bond with unwanted poisons, minerals in the soil. The same is true for spinach. If spinach or leeks are growing in contaminated soil their iron picks up the contaminants. I never eat spinach unless I grow it myself, or my friends do. For more on this topic, see Wilhelm Pelikan's *The Secrets of Metals*.

Another favorite of the French which I also love is hazelnuts. I remember going for walks with one of my aunts in Burgundy where we were sent for little vacations so my mother could have a rest from her three lively daughters. We used to eat the hazelnuts from the bush that I was allowed to climb. I like to make hazelnut-chocolate spread. You can buy hazelnut butter and then add organic dark chocolate powder and mix it with honey. Children love it, and it contains iron, as well.

leeks	41 mg. iron
millet	9 mg. iron
spinach	6.6 mg. iron
hazelnuts	5.0 mg. iron
dried peaches	6.5 mg. iron

The French do not have the enormous obesity problem that the people in the United States have. They have not disconnected themselves entirely from the process of growing foods. However, they do have a problem with alcoholism that causes many deaths and suicides. I lost one of my French cousins to this terrible affliction.

What is not lost in Europe in general is the appreciation and celebration of food. They acknowledge its importance by serving it artistically and making eating a joyful experience rather than just throwing foods in one's mouth. They take the time to enjoy their food, whether they are Italians, Spaniards, French, Dutch, or Norwegians. Eating in Europe is a celebration. Sometimes it goes beyond enjoyment into gluttony, sensuous eating, living to eat, but that is not the norm. This celebration must be part of a family's habit. Then the food will become a way to enjoy each other's company and reconnect. Under no circumstance should a family eat while watching television.

One wonderful way to learn about food and collect great recipes is to go to a bookstore and browse in the cooking section. Cookbooks are marvelously entertaining and provide a source of inspiration to new cooks, or experienced ones wanting to try out new things. I remember my mother had bought a new very fat cookbook when we lived in Annaba, Algeria, and for months my parents were busy in the kitchen making all sorts of cakes with wonderful decorations and other new recipes. It was a feast for us kids because my parents were having fun experimenting in the kitchen.

The Mediterranean landscape offers the southerners a wonderful opportunity to cook with herbs. The scent of thyme, rosemary, lavender, dill, and marjoram is never very far from Italian or French kitchens. Spain is a bit behind in that respect, with the exception of some cities such as Barcelona. I walked through much of Spain, day after day, in fields of lavender and thyme, but what I was served for food was white rice, a piece of fish, and caramel pudding with no herbs at all. The Italians and the French are the experts in the use of herbs. Herbs are a very important part of the diet. In my large gardens in Wisconsin, I have grown all sorts of herbs and cannot do without them in my cooking. They add beauty to taste all year long, as one can easily dry them for winter's use.

> Seasonings have come into increasing use the more human development has enabled us to come into full possession of our body and experience it in all its inner differentiation. In Egyptian times, spices were used only by priest-kings. Later, royal courts followed suit. In the great days of Greece and Rome, they came into general but moderate use. The spice trade became a considerable business, especially in the hands of the Arabs. Spices commanded a very high price in the Middle Ages. Pepper, for example, came to play a role similar to that of gold. It was often used in place of money. Pepper customs were set up at borders, and kings and princes made each other presents of pepper....
>
> Wherever the enhancement of consciousness was made to serve a sharper development of thought and concept, there were seasonings in the food and on the table.... The shift from a dream state of mind to full sensory alertness, such as was now required for observation of the laws of nature, meant preparing and developing the body for this task.

A thorough study of seasoning agents shows that they occupy the halfway point between food and medicine.[38]

Kitchens should therefore contain a variety of seasonings, and cooks become artists at blending them in an "aromatic symphony"....

All this indicates the close ties between seasonings and heightened awareness—not only on the part of the cooks but also for those who eat the food they season. Awareness is sharpened by its flavor and aroma, and the more subtly the sense of taste has been aroused, the greater the interest that follows the food through the digestive process. We see what an awakening has taken place, even physiologically, and how a true art of spicing helps digestion by rousing a person's livelier participation.[39]

When cooks are in the kitchen, they become "magicians who take care of family needs, depending on the season, the occasion, and the people for whom the food is prepared. Here Dr. Hauschka's indications are priceless and full of wisdom:

Melancholics do well to relieve their body-bound heaviness of soul with the choleric spices: pepper, paprika, curry, mustard, and the various radishes.... Hot-blooded cholerics should, however, avoid hot sauces, and turn instead to seasonings of a more melancholic trend. They need solid, formative, mineralizing root forces to tame the sulfur forces that rule their metabolisms. Bitter or salty roots and bark just fill the bill [salt, caraway, summer savory, lovage, cinnamon, wormwood, gentian root]. Phlegmatic persons, on the other hand, are too much involved in their own psychological processes (i.e., their life bodies). It is good for them to let the sanguine seasonings lend them wings, or the choleric ones rouse them. Onions, chives, and *Umbeliferae* [coriander, fennel, caraway, and anise] should be included in their diet, along with flavorings in the sharp category [pepper, paprika, leeks, horseradish, mustard]. The sanguine tendency to be emotionally scattered and torn in all directions needs such phlegmatic foods as nuts, olives, and

---

38 Hauschka, *Nutrition*, p. 110.
39 Ibid., p. 111.

almonds. And the herb lovage has a calming and settling effect. A vegetable diet is always helpful, too, in holding the sanguine metabolism to concentrated effort, which in turn means better mental concentration.[40]

Italy was the home of the Renaissance, France of the Enlightenment, and herbs have much to do with both. All is not in the intellect. We can see that with this knowledge one can go a long way in taking care of the family and, just as important, learning about ourselves, the bounty of nature, and the wisdom behind it.

I cannot omit the wonderful chestnut which is part of the diet in Europe. It is sold in the winter by street vendors on busy street corners in Paris or Florence. To make a delightful dessert, one cooks them in boiling water, peels them, and puts them in the blender with water or cream, sugar, and vanilla. One can also buy the wonderfully rich chestnut sweet puree that comes in jars like jam and is served on ice cream. The chestnut tree is a beautiful tree in spring with its great spiral-like flowers and in the autumn with its rich brown chestnuts. It is full of minerals and other nutrients that are excellent for children and nursing mothers.

LAND OF SWEETS

It was mentioned earlier that the Far Eastern countries have a diet that is much less sweet and more "mineral-salt" than the Western world, which includes Europe and the Americas and is more inclined toward sweets. The predominance of sugar in the diet has grown to tremendous proportions. I was in Russia a couple of years ago, and the number of cafés with exquisite sweets and cakes of all kinds was phenomenal. These places were packed with delighted customers young and old, families and students, all enjoying coffee and hot chocolate with plenty of cake. It seemed they could not get enough

---

40 Ibid., p. 113.

sweets, and they are catching up with their neighbors. We should study this phenomenon and gain insight into our Western society.

Sugarcane originally came from Malaysia, and later India; it then went to the Middle East, which developed refinements in the realm of sugar, honey, and date sugar, and these were brought to the West through the Crusades and other invasions. One can experience this by walking in any old city's bazaar in the Middle East. Their sweets and creative arrangements for their displays are unequaled anywhere else in the world. We have inherited the knowledge and technology of sugar products, developed further by the discovery of sugar beets. Let us look at a brief and simple history of sugar consumption.

> The conquests of Alexander brought a new development with them. When Alexander led his armies through Persia to India, the Greeks came upon "a reed that brings forth honey unaided by bees." This was the sugar cane already then under cultivation in India. Its culture spread through Persia to Egypt and soon became known to the whole civilized world of the period. It was the Arabs who discovered how to crystallize its sap and carried on a highly developed sugar business. The boiled sap was poured into cones made of palm leaves, thus creating the original sugar loaves.
>
> Charlemagne did much to further the Eastern spice trade, and this included sugar. Then the crusades helped to spread the European use of sugar. Columbus took sugar cane to America, and thus gave rise to the sugar plantations that now occupy eighty percent of the arable land of Cuba.
>
> Sugar remained a luxury, however, through the greater part of the Middle Ages. It was only in comparatively recent times that Frederick the Great, Maria Teresa, and Joseph II, those "enlightened despots," decreed that sugar was to be regarded as a food, whereupon they eased its importation by lowering duties and taxes on it....
>
> About 1800, the German scientist F. A. Achard discovered that sugar beets contained exploitable amounts of sugar. It took

another twenty years to breed beets with enough sugar in them to warrant their production on a commercial scale.[41]

The passage of time has meant a gradual descent from the blossom to the stem, then to the root:

Blossom	Honey	Time of the Patriarchs
Stem	Cane sugar	Alexander the Great
Root	Beet sugar	Napoleon

From the standpoint of shape, material, and function, the blossom, stem, and root are three clearly distinguished portions of the plant. They belong together as three parts of an organism. But each of the parts is designed to perform one distinct function....

Honey is the product of cosmic influences in the plant. And the life lived in the times of the patriarchs was equally permeated by impulses that came directly from the spiritual world into human wills. There was as yet no such things as personal will and personal concepts. Individuality was still undeveloped.

Central Europe was undergoing its consolidation in the cane sugar period. Cities were being built up; efforts were being made to introduce some social order and sense of belonging into the conglomerate of peoples, and everyday life was deeply permeated by religion. All this indicates that feeling was then the guiding principle.

Then came our time, a period when thinking seems as deeply immersed in things of Earth as the sugar beet is deeply rooted in the soil. Present-day thought is in this sense rootlike. In our time, the word's affairs are governed by intellect and reason....

Honey is harvested virtually without the use of technology. In the Middle Ages, with its palm-leaf molds, cane sugar production, too, was still very close to nature. But beet sugar production is based on very complex technological devices.

Thus we see a change in the state of human consciousness going hand in hand with changes in human eating habits. The example sugar presents is but one of many....

---

41 Ibid., pp. 62–63.

One of Rudolf Steiner's most impressive discoveries was that of the relationship of thinking, will, and feeling to the threefold structure of the body as the physiological basis of human soul life. According to this, thinking rests upon the nerve and sense organism, feeling on the rhythmic system, will on the limbs and metabolism....

Now if it is true that human beings are related to the threefold plant...this fact has important consequences for nutrition. Honey, cane, and beet sugar have a stimulating effect on the corresponding body parts: the metabolism [honey], the rhythmic system [sugar cane], and the nerve-sense organism [beet sugar]....

Sugar is in this sense a food that strengthens the soul and gives it a wholesome "I"-awareness. It enhances personality....

	1903	1914
England	46.4	40.8
United States	32.0	33.6
Switzerland	20.7	34.0
France	20.1	17.7
Germany	19.5	34.1
Australia	10.6	17.0
Russia	6.7	13.3

Sugar consumption per capita in kilograms
(Ulmann's Encyclopedia of Technological Chemestry)

The Western world, with its strongly developed individualism and intellectuality, consumes sugar in quantities many times greater than the East, where...the old patriarchal systems remain.[42]

This extensive quote shows trends over several thousands of years, trends that correlate with humanity's evolution of consciousness. We are meant to use our thinking ability, and our English-speaking world is the leader in this endeavor. The sugar consumption of

---

42 Ibid., pp. 62–66.

England, the United States, and Germany far surpasses that of other countries. The personality cult, the selfish ego, is linked with the high consumption of sugar. When we eat sweets we become more aware of our distinct self; we feel the luxury of selfhood. We come into our own as opposed to getting lost in our surroundings. Russia as it is emerging from its devastating experience with communism is gradually coming into individuality and personality, and slowly but surely lovely warm cafés are popping up everywhere to awaken within the Russian psyche the birth of individuality, a new feeling of being comfortable with one's self.

Now it is up to individuals to choose what kind of sugar they want to use, whether they want to affect the brain and nervous system (sugar beets), or the metabolism (honey), or breathing (sugar cane). Corn, syrup, and fig syrups, as well as many new sweets, are now available, but people can look at the picture of the threefold plant, with the human threefold nature, and decide what they want.

We are becoming a global society and I sincerely feel that across our planet sugar consumption is rising, because people everywhere are being called to become individuals. Trendy cafés are everywhere, and young people are demanding such places where they can interact, meet others, and enjoy being alone with their sweet beverages and, of course, their laptop computers.

It is a wonderful trend which I thoroughly enjoy whether I am in Iceland, Morocco, Jerusalem, Istanbul, Tunis, Marrakesh, Madrid, St. Petersburg, Delhi, Bangkok, Portland, New York City, or Beijing. Youth are everywhere, bringing new impulses into all these various societies, and sugar has a lot to do with it.

Along with the rise in sugar consumption is the rise of diabetes. One must learn to use sugar sparingly, so as not to overburden the digestive system. If we can provide out bodies with a slow release of sugar through eating carbohydrates, then we do not shock our system with instant sugar. Eating more fresh and dried fruits, cereals, grains, honey, and whole grain bread will provide all the sugar we

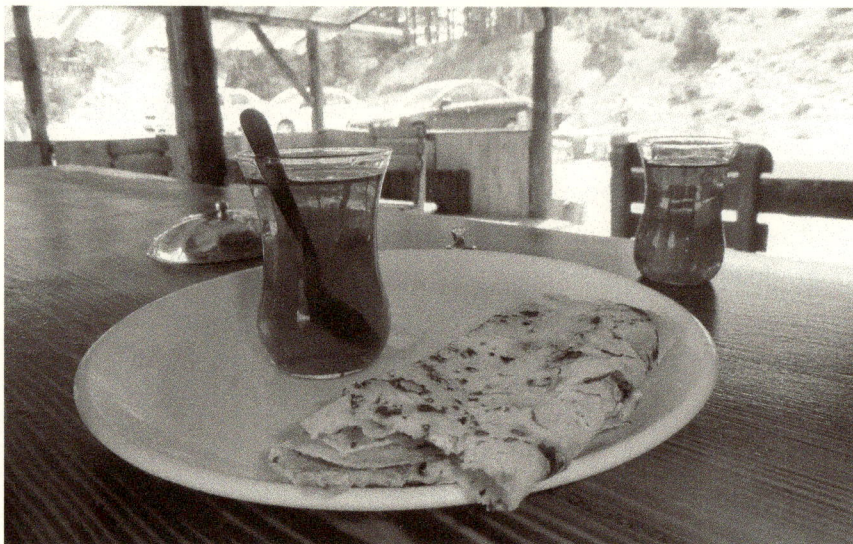

A delightful snack in the mountains along the western coast of Turkey, freshly made by women sitting on the ground

need—slow sugar as opposed to the shock of white sugar or refined white flour.

> The human personality can reveal itself through sugar. "Where sugar arises, the 'I'-organization appears in order to orient the subhuman (vegetative and animal) corporeality toward the human being." In this regard, people reverse the plant-formation process and overcome the animal process by consuming sugar. Sugar, therefore, mediates "a kind of innocent 'I'-consciousness"; it endows human beings with a natural personality character....
>
> One might ask about the possible causes of this almost unbelievable increase in sugar consumption (in the Western world). We may conjecture that the evolution of modern humankind, with its overly intense and one-sided development of personality, leads people to search unconsciously for support in the physical realm. People thus succumb to a kind of addiction that forces them to eat more and more sugar for the same effect. A pathological condition has long since come about that has been impressively diagnosed today. And there is yet another error with serious consequences stemming from the fact that sugar consumption makes possible and

stimulates the development of the human forces of consciousness. However, if people do not do this—if they do not sufficiently use the instrument thus prepared—development in a false direction takes place....

Rudolf Steiner describes a new polarity that exists between those who eat a lot of sugar and those who eat little. Those who use little sugar, "they are the weak peoples with regard to physical strength"; the others are the "strong peoples." Is this not another indication of the primeval polarity between Eastern and Western peoples? In the East, sugar is used more moderately, but in such a way as to best further spiritual forces. In the West, people develop their forces much more in the earthly spheres, in the physical world.... Food that has carbohydrates gives the body forces that it needs for work, movement....

Steiner wrote...when I chop wood—when I apply force externally—I become weak. But if a force is built inwardly in me that can transform carbohydrates into sugar...then I become strong.

This expresses what Rudolf Steiner called "the secret of humankind.... The point is not that one is filled up by food, but rather that food develops forces within the body." Food can do this only if it contains such forces itself—and it is just these forces that have been stripped from refined sugar....

People must produce glucose from cane sugar, to the extent that they can still exert their own forces in this production. Above all, they must convert starch into sugar. In addition, Steiner said that "wheat, rye, and so on have carbohydrates in them in such a form that human beings can produce sugar in a favorable way. Actually, people can make themselves as strong as possible by means of carbohydrates.[43]

Honey is a sacred, special food. Rudolf Steiner devoted a whole lecture cycle on bees that I strongly recommend to the reader. I will only mention this passage addressed to young couples:

---

43   Schmidt, *The Essentials of Nutrition*, pp. 162–164.

Basically, it is truly a wonderful thing that such small creatures exist that are capable of extracting from blossoms, flowers, and plants that substance which they transform into this extraordinarily healthy honey, a substance that could play a more important role in human nutrition than it does today. All that is necessary is that people gain a thorough insight into how terribly important honey is as a food. For example, if it were possible to exert more of an influence on the entire field of what I might call "social" medicine, I would consider it an extremely favorable influence if couples, during the time of their engagement, would eat honey as a preparatory activity before having children. For in this way they would not have rickety children, because there is in honey a force that can affect the reproductive power in human beings, who then, in turn, transform this honey power further so as to give the offspring a proper bodily form. The parents'—more specifically, the mother's—consumption of honey has a beneficial effect that extends itself to the bony, skeletal frame of the child.[44]

Honey is also excellent for older people, who should decrease their intake of milk and take in more honey instead. When I am traveling for any length of time or walking long distances, I carry my own jar of honey and a thermos so I can have my daily allowance of this very precious food with tea. It gives me great endurance and strength. I don't go without it. I buy honey from the locals wherever I am, and in Wisconsin I have my own bees and extract my own honey, which is extremely rich because I have planted special herbs which they love. Thyme seems to be their favorite, along with melissa, the mints, anise, hyssop, marjoram, rosemary, sage, and all varieties of flowers and orchards.

Sugar and "I"-strengthening reminds me of what this "I"—this higher ego, the "I" that lives in the warmth of our body—is meant to do. Perhaps this immense craving for sweetness and the recognition that warmth and light, which we must have in the form of

---

44 Steiner, *Bees*, pp. 90–91.

carbohydrates, sugar, and sweetness, has another element to it. The following words speak also of warmth and light. These words are sweet words, food for the soul. As sugar, honey brings warmth and sweetness, and so does prayer:

> The mood of prayer brings us, on the one hand, to look at our strictly limited "I," which has worked its way from the past into the present and shows us clearly how very much more there is in us than we have put to use; on the other hand, it brings us to look toward the future and shows us much more can flow from the future into our "I" than it has grasped so far. If we realize what our soul is expressing, then in the very prayer itself we will find the strength that takes us beyond ourselves. What is prayer other than the process of lighting up in us of the very force that seeks to transcend what our "I" is at the moment? And if the "I" is gripped by this striving, it already has within it the strength to progress. If the past has taught us that we have more within us than we have ever put to use, then prayer is a cry to the divine that it may fill us with its presence....
>
> We can do the same with prayer directed toward the future. If we are anxious and afraid of the approaching future, we lack the attitude of submission that prayer can bring. We must never forget that our destiny is ordered by the wisdom of the world. A sincerely submissive mood works quite differently from anxiety and fear; whereas these hinder our development, submission enables us to approach the future with life-enhancing hope and an openness to receive it. Therefore, that submission, although it may seem to diminish us, is a powerful force carrying us toward the future so that the future enriches our souls and lifts our development to ever new heights. We have now grasped what an effective force prayer is. And realizing that this has the effect of promoting "I" development, we shall not need to expect any particular external effects, for we now know that prayer is itself a source of light, and warmth—light, because we set the soul free in relation to the future and dispose it to accept whatever may emerge from that unknown realm, or warmth, because we recognize that, although we failed in the past to bring the divine element to fruition in our

"I," we have now brought it into our feelings so that it can be an effective force in us.[45]

| prayer | past | inner warmth |
| prayer | future | inner light |

So, perhaps instead of grabbing some dark chocolates, we might just read these few words, which will provide "heavenly" effects. And then have the chocolates.

Now, in this corner of the far north, it is around 3:00 p.m.—the time of day for a coffee and chocolate break after being at work since 7:30 a.m. The liver's sugar has reached its lowest level; it reached its highest level at 3:00 a.m., when it was full of sugar, so now is the time to replenish.

PERSIA

Persia now comes to mind with its wonderful diet of rice, lamb, exquisite melons, pomegranates, citrus, dates, cucumbers, eggplant, greens, feta cheese, healthy flat breads, raisins, walnuts, and almonds. The Persians are generous like all the Middle Eastern people. Their parties and festivals include massive amount of foods: subtly flavored saffron rice dishes cooked with pieces of lamb, cumin dishes, stewed soups with chickpeas and lamb, cinnamon or rose scented sweets, and beautiful sienna-colored tea.

A famous dish which everyone enjoys in Persia is eggplant cooked with meat and served on a bed of rice. Eggplant is a loved vegetable throughout the Middle East. It is cooked and mashed with yogurt or chickpeas and served with bread for snacks or as part of a meal.

The eggplant belongs to the nightshade family, a family of poisonous plants that includes belladonna, henbane, thorn apple, nicotiana, the famous potato, and tomato. Eggplant, like the other members of the family, contains much nitrogen. Let us learn more about

---

45 Steiner, *Transforming the Soul*, vol. 2, p. 74.

poisonous plants and why they are so attractive to us sometimes. What is it that they *do*? Again, this is a bit complex, but well worth plowing through. We know proteins are made up of nitrogen (N), oxygen (O), hydrogen (H) and carbon (C).

Now what is it that makes plants poisonous? It is plant protein, the same substance normally produced in seeds when plants are fructified by the animal sphere, but—in the case of poisonous plants—protein that has been denatured through too deep a penetration by the animal nature. When plants go beyond what is plantlike and take over formative processes that properly belong only to the animal realm, there is a corresponding depression of the life-element in the protein formed. Protein is always broken down by a development of conscious feeling and autonomous motion; consciousness is always achieved only at the expense of purely vegetative life. That is why, for instance, nerve substance cannot be regenerated. But protein breakdown is a normal function of the animal body. In the plant where it is abnormal, it produces poison.

Now what happens when the life-giving elements, oxygen and hydrogen in the form of water, are removed from protein? If no remnant of life remains, the result is cyanide....

Now a slow stepwise breakdown and suppression of life-elements takes place in poisonous plants and this process generates the whole list of plant poisons in substances ranging from protein to cyanide.

Protein	C H O N	7 11 2.5 2
Caffeine	C H O N	7 9 2 3.5
Atropine	C H O N	9 .5
Morphine	C H O N	7 8
Strychnine	C H O N	7
Nicotine	C H N	7 10 1.5
Cyanide	C N	7

These few examples serve to show the degeneration that takes place between normal protein stage and cyanide, the deadliest of poison. This poison-forming process is a gradual dying, especially when animal protein is used as a basis of comparison.

What happens to animal protein when life leaves it? It becomes carrion. The substances this process forms are called ptomaine poisons. They are very closely related to plant poisons.[46]

I mention the eggplant because it is very much part of the diet of the Middle East. In that respect, the region has so much sunlight that a diet which includes these nightshade plants such as the eggplant does no harm. They have so much light that a bit of darkness can be absorbed, and perhaps it actually brings us more consciousness. I will mention this poisonous plant activity in more detail later and from another angle.

> Potatoes and tomatoes may be viewed as foods that help the consciousness soul take its first baby steps, because they stimulate the head's intellectual activity and bolster a certain egoistic self-satisfaction.[47]

In Persia people have not lost sight of "cooking as a science." The people often munch on sunflower seeds. Sesame seeds are made into a butter or oil, so the people have remarkably strong teeth. Because they live on a high plateau, well above sea level, Persians have wonderfully developed lungs. As Indo-European people they are well-proportioned, and the men and women are known for their physical beauty.

Tea is a national drink, but with just sugar and no milk. In the bazaar the samovar adopted from Russia is always brewing some. The *chai khune* tea houses are part of the Middle Eastern scene, where men come for socializing and talk politics or play a game of backgammon. This is a scene that is common from one end of the Middle East to the other. Newspapers are read, loud conversations heard, and tempers irrupt when there are arguments.

---

46 Hauschka, *The Nature of Substance*, pp. 81–82.

47 Hauschka, *Nutrition*, p. 104.

Tea is grown on vast plantations on the shore of the Caspian Sea where I spent a summer with my two-year-old son while his father was serving in a field hospital dealing with horribly wounded victims from the Iraq–Iran War.

Tea is served as a welcoming drink to guests in small glasses with crystal sugar in a small bowl along with sweets. I grew to love this beverage, which I had tasted for the first time at age four or five when I stayed over regularly with an aunt in Burgundy and she served it to me with milk and sugar.

> [Unlike coffee drinking,] tea causes a loosening of the life body from the physical.... The physical body is not felt to be on a solid footing. Rather, one has the opposite experience of feeling its wise structure out of reach and deserted while the life body's fluctuating tides take over and influence one's thought life. Thoughts become harder to hold together and cannot attach themselves so easily to facts. Fantasy is stimulated to the point of seeming brilliance that can readily degenerate into a mere display of mental fireworks.
>
> Tea drinking makes thought witty, light, and scintillating. These qualities are typical of a certain phenomenon today, and we can easily see why tea has been called "the drink of diplomats."[48]

More about tea

> Consider diplomats. If one thought joins another, if one thought comes out of another, that's bad for them. When diplomats are logical, they are boring. They must be entertaining. In society people don't like to be wearied by logical reasoning—"in the first place" ... "second" ... "third"—and if the first and second were not there, the third and fourth would, of course, not have to be thought of! A journalist cannot deal with anything but finance in a finance article. But if you are a diplomat you can be talking about nightclubs at the same time that you're talking about the economy of a certain country, then you can comment on the cream-puffs of Lady So-and-So, then you can jump to the rich soil of the colonies,

---

48 Ibid., p. 117.

after that discuss where the best horses are being bred, and so on. With a diplomat one thought must leap over into another. So those who must to be charming conversationalists follows their instincts and drink lots of tea.

Tea scatters thoughts; it lets one leap from one to another. Coffee links one thought to another. If you must leap from one thought to another, then you must drink tea. And one even calls them "diplomats' teas."[49]

The family is the center of the Persian lifestyle, as in other Moslem countries. I remember one party in someone's garden in the northern part of Iran where I was living alone with my son. I had been invited by a wonderful warm lady to her home, and we ate a memorable meal which included a bed of rice and a mixture of crushed walnuts cooked in a pomegranate concentrate sauce with lamb. Then there was tea with sweets and fresh walnuts from her garden. We then all retired to bedrolls on the ground and had a wonderful nap to the pleasant sounds of birds, insects, and water flowing through the irrigation paths in the gardens.

One of my all-time favorite breakfasts was a mixture of all sorts of fresh greens, including scallions, parsley, dill, tarragon, and radish, served on a large plate and accompanied by fresh bread from the local bakery, feta cheese, and black tea from the Caspian Sea. We ate this on the floor sitting on carpets.

The radish is a wonderful food, and the French eat it with bread, butter, and salt. In Persia, I ate it for breakfast and snacks. Let us look again at this plant:

Looking at a whole plant you have the root, the stem, the leaves, and the flower. It is a strange thing with a plant. The root down there grows very similar to the soil, especially in containing a lot of salts, and the flower up top grows very similar to the warm air. Up there it is like a continuous cooking process in the heat of the Sun.

---

49   Steiner, *From Sunspots to Strawberries...*, p. 112.

The flower therefore contains oils and fats, especially oils. Looking at a plant we thus have salts being deposited below. The root is rich in salts, the flower in oils.

The consequence is that when we eat the root we get many salts into our gut. These salts find their way up to the brain and stimulate the brain. Salts thus stimulate the brain. And so it is quite good, for instance, for someone suffering from headaches—not migraine-like headaches but headaches that fill the head—to eat roots. You can see that many roots have a certain salty harshness. You can tell from the taste. But if you eat flowers, that is where the plant is really half-cooked already. Up there you already have the oils; that is something which above all greases the stomach and the gut; it has an effect on the abdomen.... The root of the plant is related to the head. The flower of the plant is related to the gut and so on.[50]

If you need something to stimulate your thinking, you should use the salty stimulus of radishes in particular, for instance. This will be good for someone who is not very lively in the head, for it'll get thoughts moving a bit if this person adds radishes to food....

We can say that radishes stimulate our thinking. And you need not be all that active in your thinking; eat radishes and the thoughts will come, such powerful thoughts that they will even create mighty dreams. People who eat a lot of potatoes do not get powerful thoughts; but they will get dreams that make them heavy. And people who have to eat potatoes all the time will really be tired all the time and always want to sleep and dream. Therefore, the kinds of food that are actually available to people play an important role in the history of civilization.[51]

The other wonderful meal is to take a juicy cantaloupe or other melon, split it in half, add walnuts, put a bit of honey over it, and then scoop it out. This is a nutritious breakfast as well. Children always enjoy such food. This part of the world is ideal for growing melons. During the growing season, we can see small trucks full

---

50 Steiner, *From Mammoths to Mediums...*, pp. 200–201.
51 Ibid., p. 202.

of melons driving through the city and countryside. The intense heat and the rich minerals in the earth bring out the most subtle flavors in these delicious fruits. They are refreshing, and fresh melon drinks are sold on the street corners. This is one more way for Middle Eastern people to be healthy.

Melons and cucumbers are cooling and wonderful in the hot summer. Cucumber can also be used for making facials. When you make a cuke salad just apply some extra cucumber to your face with some yogurt, wipe it off before you serve your meal, and hope no one shows up while your are cooking.

Rice is also the staple of Persia. It is served in enormous quantities, and Persians have a very distinct way of preparing it. It is steamed using a heavy lid covered with cloth so no steam will escape, and a wonderful aroma comes from the separated rice grains. People sometimes line the pan with potatoes and a bit of oil. The Persians love this bottom of the pan, and it also helps keep the rice from burning. All the qualities which were discussed regarding the Far East apply here as well. The rice diet furthers the ability to think, and Persia has exported great brain power: doctors, pharmacists, engineers, artists, and writers who have chosen to leave their land for political reasons.

Here is a favorite rice recipe for a family: two or three cups of rice, two or three potatoes cut up finely, and one-half cup or more of fresh or dried dill. Put the potatoes and dill on top of the rice, cover with water, bring to a boil, and simmer. Serve with yogurt. Dill, a plant full of light and aromatic oils, combined with the darkness of the starchy potatoes and the very light silica of the rice make it a very balanced meal. The addition of yogurt adds freshness and calcium to make a meal which unites the beings of Light and Dark.

Persia was the land of Zarathustra, a great initiate who brought the religion of light and dark to the world thousands of years ago. It was also in Persia that the breeding of plants originated, taught by wise men. All of our plants have been cultivated from two main families of fruits and cereals: the lily and the rose. The discoveries all stem from this ancient part of the world. The lily comprises onions, leeks, garlic, chives, and all the cereals. The rose family comprises all our fruits.

> All the various lilies have the six-pointed star of Zarathustra as their flower pattern. Tradition links lilies to the goddess Isis, and the so-called Madonna lily is a Christian version of the same. Lilies are the plant of wisdom....
>
> The grasses from which grains were developed are also related to the lily family.[52]

Wheat, rye, barley, and oats are the cereals that have developed from the lily family to become the staple of our diet, providing us with healthy carbohydrates.

Earth—Form	Wheat	rich in calcium salts
Water—Tone	Rye	rich in potassium
Air	Barley	rich in silicic acid
Fire	Oats	rich in magnesium salts....

The characteristics noted here make our four main grains excellent dietary aids for overcoming imbalances of the four temperaments. Melancholics take to oat confections because of warmth forces they contain.... Cholerics, the opposite of melancholics, like wheat and rye, and sometimes let themselves be weighed down by dumplings....

Lilies and the cereals related to them are...offspring of the Moon principle—the regent of wisdom and governor of nerve processes. A study of the rose, however, shows that it bears the Sun's signature.

Because of the Sun forces they embody, plants of the rose family have an entirely different relationship to earth from lilies. They even grow into very large trees....

---

52 Hauschka, *Nutrition*, p. 87.

The fruits of today are all descendants of the rose. They possess nutritive qualities very different from those of cereals in that they do not build tissue but instead help body and spirit work harmoniously together.... Fruit...nourishes our humanity by linking our physical and our cosmic being. Its effect is felt in the life of our will and moral creativity.

Fruit feeds the circulatory processes and even has a direct part in making blood itself.[53]

The lily and the rose have the same relationship as nerves and blood. The latter are kept cleanly separated, physiologically, for if they touched, illness would result. It is of prime importance that each function independently, keeping to its own set of laws, yet in harmonious cooperation with each other. It may not be at all far-fetched to remind our readers here of the English War of the Roses—really a war between the lily (the white rose) and the red rose.... It takes quite a bit of doing on a lofty level to unite the lily and the rose or to transform one into the other.[54]

The French monarchy adopted the lily as its flower, as we can see in France's museums, carvings, monuments, and castles, and the English adopted the rose. The lily is under the Moon sign, the rose under the Sun sign. We are still trying to figure things out between the French and the English, myself included.

> Lily for wisdom, Moon, nerves, thinking, grains,
> Rose, blood, Sun, action, willing, fruits.
>
> Thinking versus will;
> Feeling is where the two meet!
>
> Bread and jam,
> Bread and wine.

---

53 Ibid., pp. 89–91.
54 Ibid., pp. 92–93.

GERMANY

Oktoberfest in Germany is a national festival like the sheep festival in the Middle East, but it is as different as one can imagine. A German friend of mine who is a police officer told me stories about the festival which made me cringe. He said that after the festival is over, along with all the throwing up that too much drinking brings about, he with his coworkers have to carry unconscious people out of the halls where the celebration is taking place. People pass out and remain there until someone moves them. He told me these tales as if it was perfectly acceptable to behave thus. This is in central Germany, but it happens countrywide. I saw many beer gardens there. They provide a favorite place for the German public to relax and spend the evening with friends, socializing after a long day at work. I do not drink, so I had to have a drink of fizzy water with apple juice in order to not look too conspicuous and out of touch.

I enjoyed Germany and would happily make it my home because I felt very comfortable living in a society that closely resembles the United States. The people are hardworking, serious, self-motivated, and they love beer.

When I first experienced Oktoberfest in Stuttgart I was twenty-three and enjoyed the universal festive mood. In France we did not have this massive display of liveliness. There celebrating is more of a family affair, entertaining friends in one's home rather than the whole town involved in a public brawl. The French go to the market, then go home and enjoy their meals and friends in seclusion, or they go to the cafés instead of beer gardens. To me it was a welcome change to see people partying in hordes in public.

Germany is a country of forests, meadows, rich valleys, rivers, and farmland at the center of Europe, bounded by the North Sea on one side and Rhine River. The former inhabitants were the wild Germanic tribes that celebrated with nature festivals during the year. Collot d'Herbois once told me that they are all lumberjacks.

I see Oktoberfest as a remnant of those old celebrations. Everyone loosens up with the spirit running in their veins, and they experience a bit of the old aliveness. The materialistic trend is taking its tolls on the German psyche; its deadening intellect needs to get shaken up by these wild nature festivals. For a few hours people are allowed to be more than thinking machines, and they actually feel alive, thanks to the alcohol. That is what it appears to be, but is it something else? I think so.

Their diet of meat and potatoes, sausages, eggs, and creamy cakes is heavy with protein and fat. The Germans, like the Americans, have heart and ulcer problems stemming from their diets. But the Germans have dark rye bread, wonderful nutritious bread compared to the empty white-flour French baguette.

Alcohol contains neither nitrogen nor distorted proteins. It is a combination of carbon, oxygen, and hydrogen, active in ways that make it a dangerous poison for the "I." East and West offer the psyche stimulation and a blunting of one's social sensitivity. Alcohol undermines human self-mastery.

Grapes originate in Greece, and it was there that wine first came into general use. In fact, it played a ceremonial role in the mysteries of Dionysus, while the Bacchanalian rites carried wine-drinking to an excess for which we no longer understand the reason. But it is apparent that wine had a mission for that period. What sort of mission was this?

If we study the grape perceptively, we will see what a special kind of fruit it is. It produces seeds, but their germinal power is very weak. It seems as though this plant had carried its development beyond the point at which most plants stop.... Grapes pour their all into the berry....

The high point to which the grape has carried its development is the product of an energy similar in kind to the power of self-mastery with which the "I" governs the blood.

Wine's mission in the days of Greece and Rome was, then, that of laying the foundation for a new, down-to-earth, human self-awareness. Until then, consciousness had been something held in common by families and clans. A new element had to be introduced to pave the way for "I"-consciousness.

Wine had the mission of developing this in the sense that it undermined people's earlier clairvoyant wisdom. It bound blood and "I" together, so that blood became the organ of "I"-awakening. Human beings became bold and self-confident, entirely on their own and no longer dependent on outer, clairvoyantly perceived guidance.... Old clairvoyant perception of spiritual reality was to be uprooted and destroyed in preparation for developing the brain as the instrument of the "I."[55]

To take alcohol now is to produce a counter-"I" in oneself. It has the effect of influencing action that should spring freely from the resolution of the "I"; alcohol thinks, feels, and acts in place of the "I." People in this situation allow a purely external, material "I" to dictate to them. Alcohol prevents their "I" from acting, thus making them its slave.

It will be clear from the preceding that for a truly striving spirit to take alcohol at all is retrogressive. It closes the doors one was about to open. For habitual takers, there is also the problem of physical undermining. It is only a small step from mental confusion and the unleashing of violent feelings to circulatory disturbances accompanied by exhaustion. And then comes the hangover with the depositing of uric acid in the head that goes with too fast and disordered a circulation. The poisons that should have been excreted in urine and feces are instead stored up in the brain. And the blood, too, fails to renew itself....

In addition to all this, the sufferer's reproductive glands are affected. This is particularly true for women. Male drinkers ruin their nervous system, women their ovaries.[56]

I spent two months in Tintagel, Cornwall, England, to work on a project.[57] England, Ireland, and all the northern countries like

---

55 Ibid., pp. 199–120.

56 Ibid., pp. 119–121.

57 See Valandro, *Touched*.

Germany also have high alcohol consumption. A local historian told me that certain families in Cornwall still have clairvoyance capabilities from the old days. They have dreams, visions, and premonitions which they did not ask for. They come uninvited. He said he knew of one lady who hated this capacity and drinking alcohol helped her get rid of this fearful state of mind. This corresponds with the facts that we just mentioned. So could it be that some of the old Germanic clairvoyance still needs to be discarded in order to be replaced by the development of the intellect, the "I," and that drinking alcohol helps? Or is it that people need to feel some aliveness from the spirit in a world that is mechanical, cold, and abstract? One could be alive without the use of alcohol. What appears alive is the spirit of alcohol rather than the real "I" of the individual.

Here where I now live and write, the little village is the home to many young people who every weekend come to ski and experience nature. But many of them drink profusely, as do the adults. Alcohol is still part of the initiation of youth, many times with terrible consequences. Last year a friend of mine who is an instructor was coming down the mountain late during the day. After the mountain was closed he noticed a figure in the snow. It was a young man who was so drunk he had passed out face down. If my friend had not found him he would have died. My friend and his wife took the man to the hospital where he had to stay for a week because he had so much alcohol in his system. He had fallen into a coma due to high alcohol content in his blood stream, and later he was very thankful to the instructor who found him.

For some, alcohol is a means of initiation, where they encounter their dark self and try to find the way out in which they gain control of the alcohol rather than the alcohol being in control of their "I."

One cannot talk about Germany without speaking of sauerkraut, as fermented cabbage is very much part of the German diet, along with the beer.

Lactic acid has an important physiological property that comes into play in the "acidic coat" of the skin—its disinfectant effect. It stops the growth of bacteria and works against putrefaction. Lactic acid is therefore a natural protection of the body against infection, providing a basis for one of the healthful effects of sour milk products (yogurt), as well as for sauerkraut. At the same time, lactic acid acts as a preservative of protein, fat, and carbohydrates. As a result, fermented products can be preserved. The consumption of sauerkraut has thus been called "ferment therapy." The value of pickled vegetables depends on the same factors. Foods pickled with lactic acid are easier to digest and stimulate the digestion. For ill persons with chronic constipation, sauerkraut is a medicinal food. Products with lactic acid have laxative effect and protect the intestinal flora. Sauerkraut, especially, is high in calcium, potassium, and magnesium and is thus antagonistic to sodium. It is thus a diuretic and works against inflammation. Therefore, it is a good food for those with arthritis and kidney or heart diseases—though it should be made without table salt. It also supports detoxification of the liver. These few indications point to the great significance of lactic acid—and the entire fermenting process—for and within human beings.[58]

Cabbage is a staple of Russia and all of Eastern Europe. It is a vegetable that is easy to grow well into the cold winter weather, and it brings warmth to the body. It belongs to the family of the crucifers, a large family of plants that I have often grown in my gardens. It comprises turnips, kohlrabi, white cabbage, red cabbage, savoy cabbage, kale, brussels sprouts, broccoli, and cauliflower. This family of plants has within itself the sulfur process, which one can distinctly smell when one is cooking it. So as a bearer of sulfur these plants are warming, the reason why one sees them often in very cold countries. The sulfur content warms us up, as do radishes, mustard, cress, and horseradish, all part of this hot sulfur family.

---

58 Schmidt, *The Essentials of Nutrition*, p. 253.

In sea water, along with magnesium, we find sulfur in the form of magnesium sulphate. This gives some idea of the enormous amount of sulfur dissolved in the various seas and oceans.

Free sulfur has been attributed to volcanic action.... To trace the origin of sulfur is to have described its being: it is a substance with a great affinity to warmth. It is inflammable, burning with a very hot, dark flame. It combines readily with the warmth-bearer, hydrogen, making hydrogen sulphide. This is a gas released by putrefactive process, with the characteristic odor of rotten eggs.... It possesses the capacity for change that we find it in six to seven modifications...that can exist within a comparatively narrow range of temperature. One form can be changed into another simply by heating....

Chemically speaking sulfur is the most active of all substances. It does not act in any one clear direction as do the halogens and oxygen; rather it forms combinations in a sociable way, creates new possibilities and supplies warmth, acting toward other substances as a kind of cook.

Sulfur's function in protein is of just such a nature. Its liking for the colloidal state and thus for everything alive, its capacity for change, and its brood warmth make it a natural mixer of substances, particularly the organic. It is the carrier of vital formative forces. Sulfur is rather a uniting force that prompts cosmic essences to work together in building up matter. It gives itself over wholly to organic life, promotes its physical functioning, and in this way keeps it clear of infringements from the side of consciousness.[59]

Could it be that sulfur is the sanguine mineral? Redheads and blond people have sulfur in their system in abundance, and it makes them choleric and sanguine, characteristics which we are attracted to. Sanguines flutter about from one thought to another like hummingbirds, never staying too long anywhere, or on any topic, and certainly don't go into depth about anything. The fiery choleric has angry outbursts that come like a flash of lightening, clearing the

---

59 Hauschka, *The Nature of Substance*, pp. 152–153.

atmosphere. The sulfur in their characters takes over and makes room for change. As a blonde with a touch of the choleric and sanguine within me, sulfur is no stranger to my character.

The herb yarrow has sulfur in it and so does chamomile. Because of the sulfur in my blond, blue-eyed constitution, when I drink a tea made of yarrow or chamomile I get a headache. My system cannot tolerate more yarrow, so I stay away from those herbs and leave them to those with a phlegmatic temperament.

I love horseradish and in August I make a paste, putting the roots right into the blender with my own vinegar and I use this mixture in the winter with cheese sandwiches, in order to fight the common head cold.

The use of these vegetables is a godsend to a diet of meat and potatoes, such as the central European diet. It counteracts the heaviness of the meat and helps with digestion, especially with the sluggish digestive system of meat eaters, and it has a "quickening effect on lazy metabolism and frees the nerve process in the head." It also helps a congested liver.

> Horseradish in particular has a distinct relationship to warmth processes that take place in the liver, in the secretion of gall. It relieves congestion in this area and helps the "I"-forces do their work of stimulating the necessary fire processes of the metabolism. This eases the nervous system and helps overcome any tendency to migraine that may exist.[60]

Here is one more lovely picture of sulfur, which all gardeners partake in:

> When we walk through the blossoming meadow in June, the month during which the Sun is in the constellation Gemini, we can feel the sulfuric element rampant in all the sprouting and flowering of nature. The soul of nature slumbers like the Sleeping Beauty amid

---

60 Hauschka, *Nutrition*, p. 99.

all this burgeoning vegetation. In their blossoms, plants come into touch with the soul sphere, the source of consciousness in animals, but with the aid of sulfur activity within them they keep the soul sphere from penetrating more deeply into their organisms. Otherwise, they would become poisonous.[61]

We can see that this large family of crucifers, meaning cross, gives much to humanity, sulfur being one of its warming substances.

"Give us this day our daily bread" is something Germans take very seriously. They must have this healthy rich dark bread in their diets using rye flour. The grains that grow in central Europe are wheat, oats in the north, barley, and rye. We know they give us carbohydrates (carbon-oxygen-hydrogen), providing us with starches, proteins, oils, and salts as they grow under the Sun's influence.

Wheat, rye, barley, and oats are the grains known and grown in Central Europe. They are wind pollinated, meaning that air currents rather than insects do the work of pollination. Cosmic soul-being, active in the atmosphere and in bees, butterflies, and other insects, touches plants, and they respond with a glorious wealth of color.[62]

Wheat has the most compact form of all the cereals, while oats with their loose arrangement of berries and the radial formation of their starch kernels grow in a way reminiscent of rice.[63]

Cereal	Protein	Fats	Carbohydrates	Salt
Wheat	10%	1%	75%	Ca
Rye	11%	2%	70%	K
Barley	12%	3%	69%	SiO_2
Oats	13%	6%	67%	mg[64]

Carbohydrates can be called "formed and fire-quickened cosmic life."

---

61 Hauschka, *The Nature of Substance*, p. 154.

62 Hauschka, *Nutrition*, p. 88.

63 Ibid., p. 89.

64 Ibid., p. 90.

Europe is part of the temperate zone of the Earth, with its four seasons giving a definite movement to the soul. Grains are marvelous foods for the human being, making it truly a food for our daily bread.

Along with dark bread, caraway seeds in many of the breads offer another very healthy combination to counteract a fatty, meat diet. This seed comes from the *Umbelliferae* (or *Apiaceae*) kingdom. It is the seed of the beautiful dill plant, which was mentioned in the Persian diet. Dill grows quite fast and displays a wealth of very intricate, fine leaves which seem to disappear into the heavens. It is one of my favorites, and it is always present in my garden. I eat it fresh in the summer sprinkled on ripe tomato slices. Dill is highly aromatic. Its family includes coriander, fennel, anise, dill, chervil, parsley, carrots, celeriac, and parsnips that all have aromatic qualities as well and are helpful when one has bloating or a sluggish digestion because of too much rich food. Including caraway seeds in dark bread will help digest a heavy meal.

With these aromatic gifts of nature we bring light into our digestion, just as the carrot with its sweet taste shows that the light process has reached deep down into the roots, the opposite signature of the potato, which is a being of darkness. These plants are beings of light and should always be in the kitchen and used in soups of all kinds, especially when using potatoes, like dill, leek, and potato soup.

> [*Umbelliferae*] begin to take effect after the liquefied food has disappeared through the intestinal wall. At this point they support the upward climb of the nutrient system. Humankind represents a continuation of the plant kingdom in the cosmic process, since we first break down the plant matter we consume, dematerialize it, and then build our own nervous system from the light forces we have freed in this way. The light that forms plants in the outer scene is the force that, when interiorized, builds the structure of the nervous system....

Umbelliferae help products that are broken down pass out of the body and help the secretion of sweat, milk, and urine, thus making room for a health-giving penetration of the physical human being by soul and spirit....

They lift, lighten, and support the upward flow of nutrients.[65]

To sum up:

The West is threatened with imprisonment in matter (potatoes, earth, darkness); the East is threatened with losing itself in formlessness (rice, light, air). Both in size and shape, the starch granules of wheat, rye, and barley show a beautiful harmony between the two polarities. The starches of Central European plants are shaped like miniature suns, even with concentric layers around their cores.[66]

MOTHER INDIA

One cannot talk about food and leave out Mother India, the home of spicy foods and completely balanced vegetarian or vegan diets based on mystery knowledge. I spent several months traveling throughout India, and have returned several times since. The last trip was a few years ago to work on a book (*Deliverance of the Spellbound God*).

I never cease to marvel at the richness of Mother India. As in all the Middle Eastern countries, there one's senses are overwhelmed by the display of spices in the marketplaces: large sacks of spices in colorful displays of gold turmeric, mustard powder, chili, paprika, cinnamon, salt, sage, thyme, savory, rosemary, and curry. All these ingredients have their place in the Hindu diet and in daily *pujda*, rituals of gift-giving at the altars of their gods. The southern meal served on large stainless steel plates is one of my favorites. It is called *tali* and involves dozens of little stainless steel bowls containing

---

65 Ibid., pp. 100–101.

66 Hauschka, *The Nature of Substance*, p. 225.

various foods: lentils or beans, vegetables, yogurt, breads, sweets, and rice. It is a true feast. I learned how to cook some of these Indian recipes to add zest to my family's diet, especially fresh *chapattis*. There are many good Indian cookbooks on the market and delightful restaurants if you are lucky enough to live near one.

The southern part of India tends to be more vegetarian, and the north allows more meat because of the Moslem population that eats meat, but both cuisines use spices extensively. When I first traveled to India in my late twenties I thought that the use of spices could be for hygienic reasons. I thought perhaps the hot spices might kill germs. I still have found no reasonable answer to why they use so many spices. It could be that the ancient Indian culture—still in its infancy in acquiring an individual "I"-force, as opposed to still being united with the world of the gods—needed a strong impetus to come down to earth. If that were the case, the heavy use of spices would do the job, making it easier for human beings to join the Earth and leave the paradise of Heaven. The spices would have the effect of rooting human beings, of making them more present on Earth and more incarnated, feeling more themselves. When we eat a hot spicy meal, we wake up a bit more; we sweat, feel the heat rising, and get red in the face. These are all symptoms of being more alive.

But that was the ancient past. Now the Hindu sages and Buddhist masters always warn their students *not* to use spices or onions in their foods, as they will disturb the meditative life. In addition to helping one feel more alive, the spices wake the lower self as well, creating havoc. Passions rise, and meditation goes out the window.

Hindus still have a very developed medical system based on old mystery knowledge. Foods are studied in terms of hot, cold, moist, and dry concepts and the constitution of the individual, as was briefly mentioned when discussing the four temperaments: choleric–fire, melancholic–earth, phlegmatic–water, and sanguine–air. India certainly has an impact on a choleric temperament such as mine.

Rice is also a staple of the Indian diet, as well as wheat *chapattis;* lentils of all shapes and colors, *dal,* provide protein for vegetarians. Lentils are part of the legume family, *Fabaceae.*

> The legumes, or *Fabaceae,* are a strange family of plants. Plants are usually exclusively vegetative and have no trace of animal characteristics or processes. Motion, which is peculiar to animals and has its physical counterpart in protein (or nitrogen), does not appear in the same way in plants, which are unable to move from place to place. Nevertheless, an element of motion enters the picture at a certain point in their development when visited by bees, butterflies, and other insects. Here the plant reaches up into the animal sphere, just as at its opposite pole, the root, it reaches down into the mineral realm. At the upper pole, we see a remarkable meeting of the living pure realm of plants, with the soul element of the cosmos, represented by the insects fluttering about them.
>
> The result of this meeting is the blossom and the seed that develops within it, producing the proteins that might be called the "shadow" cast on plants by the animal realm.[67]

> Peas, lentils, and beans are foods included in the diet because they aid the formation of proteins in the organs. They tend, as already noted with respect to excessive protein intake, to cause too much hardening, making the body tissue dense and heavy, tying body and spirit too closely together. This, plus the wholly atavistic nature of legumes, was why Pythagoras and his students avoided pulse foods. The protein they contain is more truly animal than milk.[68]

Like the richness of its religious culture, the Hindu diet is one of the most satisfying diets in my experience. Take the traditional American hamburger on a bun, with cold tasteless lettuce and fat tasteless tomatoes drenched in syrupy ketchup and compare it with

---

67 Hauschka, *Nutrition,* p. 95.

68 Ibid., pp. 97-98.

a Hindu meal, and one cannot but wonder about what is happening on the Western continent.

Part of the vegetarian diet includes coconuts. The women use coconut oil on their beautiful dark hair, along with scented jasmine flower garlands, which they use to tie up their hair. The coconut milk is used in curry sauces and in sweets and also in cosmetics and in cooking oil. The coconut tree grows along the entire eastern and western coasts of India.

When I was twenty-seven, I spent a winter in Goa where I rented a small fisherman's cabin in a coconut grove in a small fishing village where pigs roamed about, taking care of refuse. The roof and general structure of the cabin was made with palm leaves.

I spent my days on the beach watching the fishermen in their loincloths bring in their nets filled with fish. The fishermen would climb up the tall coconut trees and use sharp knives to cut down the coconuts, which I bought from them. At night they sat on the beach around a fire singing and playing simple instruments, getting drunk on the coconut liquor which drove them partly crazy. I had to be watchful at night so that they would not break down the door of my cabin.

I cooked shrimp-rice curry in earthen clay pots on an outdoor wood fire and ate coconuts. The fresh coconut juice is exquisite. It is soothing, rich, and delightfully refreshing after a day in the salty sea.

The trees' roots are shallow, barely in the soil. I always wondered how they kept themselves up. These roots are the complete opposite of the deep tap root of the pine tree, and this illustrates their origin. India was once part of a large continent called Lemuria that stretched from the islands of Malaysia all the way to Australia. It was an ancient continent that perished by fiery volcanic outbursts, much like Atlantis perished in massive floods and natural disasters of epic proportions, which we are going to reexperience in six to seven thousand years in another Ice Age.

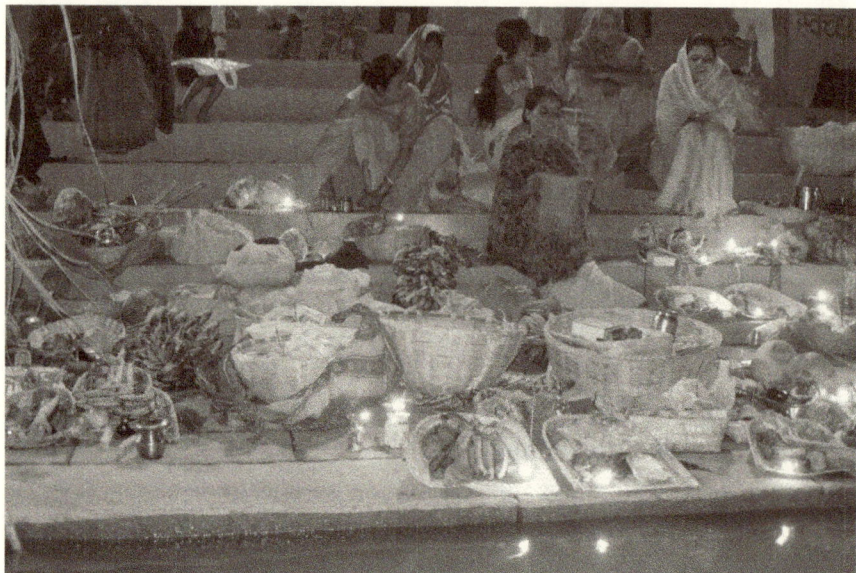

Benares, India; week end celebration on the shore of the sacred Ganges River; giving thanks with offerings to deities

That landmass called Lemuria was not as mineralized as ours, but was softer and thereby the plant life did not need to be as rooted as it does now. It was merely part of the earth. The tall coconut and other palm trees are remnants of Lemuria, although its plants were much taller than they are now.

The coconut tree grows as high as thirty meters and can reach the venerable age of a hundred years. It thrives primarily in tropical coastal regions.... Up to one hundred fruits may ripen on a tree.... Their milk has been treasured since ancient times as a refreshing, tasty drink. The fruits take fifteen months to develop in the hot tropical sun and moist tropical air. They grow as big as a human head...only the seed inside, surrounded by the nutritive "milk" contains the oil and the typical germ...the product is sixty to seventy-five percent fat and solidifies at 23° (73° F)....

The palm tree...plays a large role as a source of oil and fat. It grows to about twenty meters.... The fruit flesh provides thirty to seventy percent palm oil....

146

The aristocratic, stiff, and rigid carbon holds sway in such plants. It can produce the hardest substance—the diamond—and gives the palm leaves their formal dignity but also their inflexible shape. These plants rank fourth among the oil-producing plants in the world.[69]

If you have seen a coconut, you can attest to the strength of the fruit, which is very difficult to break open. I use a machete. The carbon strength is definitely present in these enormous fruits that come to us from another period in the Earth's history. Compared to the olive tree of the Mediterranean climate, the coconut tree is a giant gatherer of oil, fat, and sweet milk. It is a reminder of the Earth's very ancient past.

These days there is much talk of saturated and unsaturated oils. To understand them, we need to know that they have much to do with geography. The oils are made from the strong impact of the cosmic Sun forces on plant life. Depending on where we stand on Mother Earth, the rays come directly and strongly, as in the tropics, or less strongly and obliquely, as in the north:

> The activity of the cosmic forces that stimulate oil production occurs differently.... In the equatorial areas, the cosmic forces of warmth and light are absorbed at once, something that can quite typically be experienced in this warmth area. One can also say that warmth becomes earthly. The more we go northward, the more splendid do the warmth and light phenomena become. In the polar regions, warmth and light are not taken in by the earth but are radiated back. The earth acts as a reflector. It radiates back into the atmosphere. Rudolf Steiner described this phenomenon as resulting in something which gives oil formation another quality. It refers to the so-called unsaturated oleic acid. Every fatty oil has a specific oleic acid spectrum. The closer we come to the warm equatorial regions, where the forces of warmth and light become terrestrial, the more saturated oleic acid is formed by the oil-producing plants.

---

69 Schmidt, *The Essentials of Nutrition*, pp. 128–129.

It is an advantage of the oil-producing plants which grow more in the north that they can form more unsaturated oleic acid....

The closer to the skin, the more unsaturated fatty acids and the lower the melting point. The more deeply in the organism, the higher the melting point and the smaller the amount of unsaturated fatty acids.[70]

Steiner spoke of how, in the tropics, "the earth draws in the most extra-earthly" and lets the vegetation spring forth from it. Warmth and light, as cosmic forces, thereby obtain an earthly character. In contrast, these forces are most reflected back to the poles: "The Earth shines the most at the poles." Light and warmth maintain their extra-earthly character. The same holds true for mountain plants that grow at high altitudes.

The warmer it is, the more oil tropical plants produce, but their oil is more earthly. The daily rhythm rules; there are no seasons. Tropical oils exhibit more saturated oil-formation, which tends toward densification. "When the same plant can grow and flourish well in both hot and cold climates, it forms fat deposits with unsaturated fatty acids in cold climates. In warm climates, it forms deposits with saturated fatty acids." In northern regions, plants produce less oil. The warmth is radiated more strongly back into the cosmos, rather than being substantially condensed. For all that, the unsaturated fatty acid types predominate. The palm and coconut trees—with their strong, primarily saturated oil products—stand in contrast to thistle oil, rape oil, and other oils from the northern lands. In the middle, between both—in the Mediterranean—we find the olive tree. Its fruit has an oil containing seventy percent unsaturated oleic acid.[71]

Unsaturated fatty acids—north—higher melting point
Saturated fatty acids—tropics—lower melting point

Unsaturated—inflammatory—north
More active—busier

---

70 Schmidt, *The Dynamics of Nutrition.* pp. 113–114.
71 Schmidt, *Essentials of Nutrition*, pp. 126–127.

Closer to the skin—lower melting point
Too much in the diet leads to inflammation—olive—soybean

Saturated—sclerotic—tropics
Deeper in organism—higher melting point
Too much in the diet leads to sclerotic conditions—coconut—palm

So now when going shopping it will be easier to judge what it says on the bottle of oil. Will I buy coconut, olive, peanut, or grape seed oil? I use mostly olive oil, but also have many other oils for different purposes. I use them for body, hair, or face oils; salad dressing; baking; stir-frying; soups; and more. Almond, peanut, coconut, sesame: these oils are what make cooking creative, fun, and nourishing. One can also use almond oil with oil of rose, lavender, or pine as a massage or face oil, and it is inexpensive to make. I always associate the beauty of an Indian woman's hair to her use of coconut oil on it.

The Indian culture provides another asset to physical health. Spiritual life in India is still strong.[72] The older generation is very much alive, and one notices this as soon as one lands in Mother India. It envelopes a traveler with a heavy mist, a cloud of religious fervor. Living with the spiritual world, including everyday immersion in the spiritual, has its effect on the human body.

If in old age we have an interest that completely occupies our soul and spirit, something that inspires and enthuses us, it will make us youthful. The meaning of *inspiration* is that something spiritual enters the mind. Otherwise, the term would not be *inspiration* but something like *materialization*.... Being filled with enthusiasm is indeed a source of rejuvenation. Of course, we cannot prove this with rats! It is a source of rejuvenation in humans, however, and if observations in life were made in this direction, we would discover that, depending upon people's health and stamina, whatever rejuvenation could be brought about would be attained much

---

72 See, for example, Valandro, *Deliverance of the Spellbound God.*

more easily if they could be allowed sufficient time to engage in some mental activity. Mental or spiritual activity has the peculiar effect of holding together and keeping strong the glandular walls. If people are interested in keeping strong the glandular walls. If people are interested only in superficial matters all their lives, their glands and vascular walls tend to become slack more quickly than if they have an interest in spiritual and mental activities.[73]

I will end this Indian food adventure by mentioning one last delicious drink—*lassi*. It has become a big thing in the new international cuisine of the United States and Europe. Coffee shops everywhere now regularly serve these imported drinks of yogurt and fruit, but one must inquire if they are fresh and not a powdered mixture. *Lassi* drinks are part of the Indian meal, refreshing and rich. One can make them at home with yogurt and frozen fruits and serve them as snacks or as part of a meal.

LOVE AS FOOD

Let us leave the food travel realm for now and return to something mentioned a while back: the fostering of interest which makes for a healthy body. The following words for me have more sustaining value than the healthy meal of soup, bread, cheese, and avocado I ate at lunch, and one can see and feel why they work like magic on someone's soul. They can perform miracles for people who truly live by them, thereby bringing real healing forces to the human being.

> Now we can trace how an impulse from one life works into other lives—for example, the impulse of love. We can act in relation to others from the impulse we call love. It makes a great deal of difference whether we act from a mere sense of duty, convention, respectability, and so on, or from some degree of love.
> Assume that in one earthy life we are able to perform actions sustained by love—warmed through and through by love. It

---

73 Steiner, *From Comets to Cocaine...*, p. 66.

remains as a real force in our soul. What we take with us as an outcome of our actions, what is now mirrored in the other souls, returns to us as a reflected image. As we form our astral body from this, with which we descend to Earth, the love of the previous earthy life, the love that poured out and was now returned to us from other souls, is changed to joy and gladness.

Such is the metamorphosis, if we may so describe it. People do something for other human beings, something sustained by love. Love pouring from them accompanies the acts that help their fellow human beings. In passing through life between death and a new birth, this outpouring love in those lives on Earth is transmuted, or metamorphosed, into joy that flows in toward them.

If you experience joy through a human being in one earthly life, you may be sure it is the outcome of the love you unfolded toward that person in a former life. This joy flows back again into your soul during your life on Earth. You know the inner warmth that comes with joy; you know what joy can mean to us in life— especially the joy that comes from other human beings. It warms life and sustains it—gives it wings, as it were. It is the karmic result of love that has been expended.

But in our joy, we again experience a relationship to human beings who give us joy. Thus, in our former life on Earth, we had something within us that made the love flow out from us. In our succeeding life, we have the results of it, the warmth of joy, which we experience inwardly once more. And this again flows out from us. People who can experience joy in life are, again, something for their fellow human beings, something that warms them. Those who have reason to go through life without joy are different from their fellow human beings, those to whom it is granted to go through life with joyfulness.

Then, in the life between death and a new birth once more, what we thus experienced in joy between birth and death is reflected again in the many souls with whom we were on Earth and with whom we are again in our life beyond. The manifold reflected image that thus comes back to us from the souls of those we knew on Earth works back again once more.... What is it in its outcome now? Now it becomes the underlying basis, the impulse, for a quick and ready understanding of humanity and the world. It becomes the basis for the attunement of the soul that bears us along, inasmuch as we understand the world. If we find interest and take delight in the conduct of others, if we understand their conduct and find it interesting in a given earthly life, it is a sure indication of the joy in our last incarnation and of the love of our incarnation before that. People who go through the world with a free mind and an open sense, allowing the world to flow into them so that they understand it well—they have attained, through love and joy, this relation to the world.

What we do in our deeds out of love is altogether different from what we do out of a dry and rigid sense of duty.... It is the actions that spring from love that we must recognize as truly ethical; they are the truly moral deeds.[74]

Steiner goes on to explain that acts done out of antipathy, duty, or hatred will bring suffering in the life that follows, and then stupidity in the life after that, or passivity and lack of interest in the world.

As homemakers, it is important to perform our duties in the home with love for the work, love for keeping the house, love for preparing the food, love for our family and friends. The cycle must start somewhere, and the home is a wonderful beginning for such practices that, as you have seen, have far-reaching consequences. It is the beginning of leading a sacred life, to make our life sacred once more.[75] It is sacredness which comes from knowledge and not through passing fads, by copying others, or blindly following old customs. Here is an added benefit to the sacrificial work of the homemaker–mother–spouse.

A great selflessness...everything people do with intense energy, putting forth all their force and acting not on their own authority nor out of emotion—everything people do in this way gives them extraordinary strength. It is a strength that moves, so to speak,

74 Steiner, *Karmic Relationships*, vol. i, pp. 64–66.

75 See Steiner, *Start Now!* for more on this topic.

in the lower clouds of material existence, but it is, nonetheless, a spiritual force.[76]

Steiner was talking about the dedication of the Jesuits to the Pope. In my example, homemakers dedicate their work to the higher being of the family, which stands and protects them.

SOUTH AND CENTRAL AMERICA

The world of South and Central America has a special place for me. I learned Spanish when I moved to the Unites States and became friends with Colombians, Puerto Ricans, Ecuadorians, Chileans, and Mexicans. My first platonic boyfriend, whom I met when I was doing synchronized swimming in a traveling show at age sixteen, was the champion diver of Mexico. I perfected my Spanish that first summer as we traveled from one end of North America to the other, going through Newfoundland and Nova Scotia for shows in small towns, through the entire United States to the Pacific Ocean and back. My Spanish was quite good at the end of that summer, and it has been a wonderful language to know ever since. I have traveled half a dozen times to our sister continent and I love the people, the wild, diverse countries, and their ancient ways. As we have studied, the potato, tomato, and tobacco come from those lands where the ancient Aztecs and other indigenous peoples used these ingredients in their sacred ceremonies.

Their diet includes beans, rice, corn, lime, potatoes, exotic fruits, yams, avocados, onions, and a whole pharmaceutical wealth from the Amazonian region. Beans, rice, lime and corn tortillas are the staple of the Indian population. The beans provide proteins, the rice carbohydrates, and the corn and lime provide the fat.

The Indian population is short and stocky, and they have enormous strength and energy. But many villages lack simple hygienic

---

76 Ibid., vol. 8, p. 66.

habits, which invite a host of diseases. Pigs are kept near the family home in the tiny villages throughout the Andes to provide more sustenance. Water supplies are polluted, and many bronchial and skin infections as well as stomach ailments are common in these out-of-the-way villages. The wealthy population does not do much to help. Christian organizations flock to South America to preach their version of Christianity, which is not always well accepted within these Indian communities. On one trip I saw a bus-load of at least sixty kids from Maine who were spending the week building the roof on a church. They were sightseeing for a day. I thought to myself that they would have done better if they had saved the money from their travels to build latrines or a field clinic. But I have met many young American high school kids who have gone to South America to help with projects of one kind or another deep in the bush, the Amazon, or the mountains and have come back greatly changed.

I have spent much time walking in the hills and villages of Ecuador where I often heard the sound of the textile industry's weaving machines. They made clickity sounds as they created brightly colored cloth. It seems everyone had one in their home. The Indians still weave by hand as well as by machine; they have not lost their traditional arts. I visited an Indian school, and the elders there told me that the day they lose their artistic activities will be the day their people die. Their deep knowledge made them aware that they needed to keep their traditions alive by teaching young people how to weave, play musical instruments, make clothes and shoes, and knit. They wear their own distinct clothing and shoes, and the men do not cut their hair. They have traditional music that can be heard all over Europe in the subways. They also have their own diet. Those traditions, the elders said, are what they still transmit to their children in their own special schools, in order to insure that they do not die out. All the small towns have wonderful local markets once a week and regional markets where the farmers come to buy and exchange animals. These are exciting events, especially if you like photography. The colors are lively and so are the people.

South America is also the home of several of our stimulants: coffee beans, chocolate, tobacco, and coca leaves. When one walks in the Andes cocoa leaves are readily available to chew. The natives use them as a narcotic when they work in the mines or in the fields. South America is the home to the richest plant life on the planet, especially in the Amazon. Many pharmaceutical companies have taken up residence there to acquire the knowledge of the healing powers in these amazing plants and to bring it to the United States. There they transform it, patent the knowledge, and sell it back to us for enormous profits.

We spoke already about nightshade plants such as eggplants, tomatoes, and potatoes, and now we will investigate them further:

All the so-called stimulants are actually mild poisons. It is precisely their poisonous effect that enables partakers to have experiences that they could not otherwise have, or could have been achieved through considerable effort of the mind and will. The reason for this is that all stimulants affect the body's connection with the soul and spirit. The heightening or other change of consciousness that follows is experienced as pleasure or satisfaction....

Except for alcohol, poisons present in stimulants all derive from plants and are alkaloids (caffeine, theine, theobromine, nicotine).... They are produced by the cosmic soul element penetrating too deeply into the plant organism. Plants are not organized around a soul, as animals are, and the animal or soul element therefore produces a distorted protein in them. Nitrogen, which we described as soul carrier, is the protein component that makes it possible for animals to move their bodies and evokes sensation and a healthy life of instinct on the soul plane. These reactions, which are normal and healthy in animals, do not belong to the plant kingdom. This turns the soul-carrying protein element in poisonous plants into alkaloids. When these nitrogenous poisons are introduced into the human body, their chief influence is on the configuration of the soul, in the sense that they tend to derange the normal adjustment of the soul-spirit to the body. The stimuli this gives to the consciousness are relatively harmless if indulgence is not excessive and habitual, but if it is, organic damage can result.[77]

Coffee is one of the most served beverages. It seems that, from one end of the Earth to the other, people drink it in the strongest way possible. It meets the needs of modern people—it affects the thinking process.

> Rudolf Steiner has described how coffee drinking loosens the life body slightly from the physical, but in a way that still permits the physical to be felt as a solid footing. Coffee makes us more aware of our bodily structure. And since this structure is so wise and logical, our thoughts become logical in their awareness of it. Coffee thus helps thinking to find a firm foundation....
>
> Coffee is a plant that has taken up more of the soul element than is right for plants. This gives it its influence on the human soul, whose functions it takes over when it strengthens logic and coherence. This means giving continuity to the thought process.... Rudolf Steiner jokingly called coffee "the drink for people of letters." On the other hand coffee can help correct a tendency to lose the thread and stray off into inconsequential matters. However, those who want to make logic their own personal possession must avoid taking coffee and letting it do their thinking for them.[78]

As mentioned before in the chart of the alkaloids that depicts plant poisons, protein, caffeine, atropine, morphine, strychnine, nicotine, and cyanide all contain the substances carbon, hydrogen, oxygen, and nitrogen. We have seen that nitrogen carries sensation, which makes an animal and person sentient and one who feels. Nitrogen is that substance, and these poisons, protein included, all carry that element.

---

77 Hauschka, *Nutrition*, pp. 115–116.
78 Ibid., pp. 116–117.

Carbohydrates are made up of carbon, hydrogen, and oxygen, which create millions of compounds. Carbon is the form-giving substance, the carrier, and it forms the skeleton of plants. Hydrogen has a relationship to warmth and fire, and it is the earth's lightest substance, as well as having the hottest of all flames. It is an element common to all acids. We could call it the fire-substance. Then we have oxygen. It makes up 20 percent of the air, but water is 89 percent oxygen. Oxygen supports life on our planet, plant growth, sap rising, and is a source of our life from the moment we take our first breath. So in these poisonous substances the key element is nitrogen, a poison and a healing substance. Nitrogen makes up 80 percent of the air.

> Nitrogen is present in a free state only in the atmosphere. In fact, it is the carrier of air, since air is eighty percent nitrogen and twenty percent oxygen.
>
> A study of the breathing process shows that the nitrogen inhaled is exhaled, laden with moisture and carbonic acid. There is no change, neither in its composition nor in its volume. What purpose does nitrogen serve, then, if it comes out exactly as it entered?
>
> When we try to live into the movement of nitrogen flowing in and out through breathing, it can be experienced as an oscillating exchange between human and world; nitrogen moves in a pendulum-like rhythm, back and forth between the two. Thus we come to view it as the carrier of motion and rhythm, enabling oxygen to be inhaled and used air to be expelled.
>
> What would happen if there were no nitrogen in the atmosphere? We would be burned up by concentrated oxygen. The dilution of oxygen with nitrogen makes breathing and its rhythm possible....
>
> An even clearer picture emerges from a study of the movement of air currents around the Earth. The air mantle is in constant rhythmic motion. Trade winds, monsoons, and other well-known air currents are not the only phenomena of this rhythmic pattern.... Nitrogen is the carrier of this breathing as it manifests in wind, storms, and weather.

> Again, nitrogen seems inappropriately named. It should be called "movement-substance" or "air-stuff."...
>
> It is significant that nitrogen is found only in the free state in inorganic nature and never as part of any chemical compound. Because nitrogen is the carrier of movement, it cannot be bound but must remain free to move. But technology has succeeded with enormous effort in tying oxygen to nitrogen. The two substances are forced under pressure.... The result is nitric acid...nitroglycerine, and other modern explosives....[79]

I wanted to go further in talking about this substance so that we become aware of the powers living in nitrogen and the plants, which have allowed the presence of this highly powerful substance that we breathe every day. Then, when we decide to partake in coffee drinking, cigarette smoking, or ingesting other stimulants that come our way, we can understand their force. If we can make powerful explosives, then can you imagine what happens when we take in a strong cup of coffee?

When substances show their true nature, we are in awe of ourselves and the powers that reside within this very complex, perfect physical body of the human being. Then, perhaps, it will be easier to take care of this sacred temple by resisting temptations to give it to what tastes and looks good rather than what the body needs. Another aspect of taking care of this sacred temple is the fact that if we pursue some kind of spiritual practices regularly, then we automatically change our desires, needs, and wants. If we see a plate of french fries, we no longer want to eat them, and we choose what is good for us naturally without forcing it on ourselves. It is a gentle transformation that becomes a lasting one, rather than a forced relationship to food such as we experience when following proscribed diets.

If children are given the correct foods from the very beginning they will not be lured into choosing the wrong ones. When my son

---

79 Hauschka, *The Nature of Substance*, pp. 58–59.

went to college in Maine, his first year was miserable because of the food in the cafeteria. The second semester he arranged to rent a room from a couple (his former German teacher Adelheide from the Waldorf school and her husband Andreas from Holland) in their biodynamic home, and he ate good food for the next five years of his college studies.

He found that with the college cafeteria diet he just could not manage to study for the heavy class load of math, science, and engineering. The food made him sick, but with Andreas and Adelheide he had great food—their chickens, biodynamically grown vegetables, and organic meats. Andreas is famous for his breakfast based on barley and dried foods. My son also found lovely coffee shops and organic bakeries, and he proceeded to finish his studies at the top of his class.

THE LAND OF LIME AND SILICA

Now I would like to share a beautiful picture that can teach us a lot and bring certain elements of nutrition into focus. We have discussed in a variety of ways the carbohydrates made up of carbon, hydrogen, oxygen, and proteins, with nitrogen added to the other three elements. The fats and oils also contain carbon, hydrogen, and oxygen. We have mentioned the cow's relationship to oxygen, the sheep's to hydrogen, the pig's to nitrogen, the birds' to silica, and then we spoke about sugar, milk, salts, rice, poisonous substances, and various vegetables, spices, and drinks. Now this picture is one that I have enjoyed over the years while traveling, and it has helped me to understand the geography of the countries and their food. It is a picture which is often spoken of by Rudolf Steiner in many different ways.

> It is about *she and he.*
> *Silica and lime*
> *Sand and calcium*

Steiner in his agricultural course describes lime/calcium as "greedy." It draws in, it takes, and it cannot leave anything alone. The catalyzing process of lime continues until the lime is satisfied. The more you come to understand lime, the more you will call it *he*. I do not say that lime is masculine; that would give the wrong impression.

Likewise, you gradually come to call silica *she*.... You will do this because a certain affection for silica will gradually be instilled in your soul, and you will learn that silica is not greedy at all. She is also never satisfied and does not desire satisfaction. She is like a highly educated person who would never stand in the way of anything, one who has become so wise and so great that she has turned into nothing but a mirror for others. Thus you have *she*, but this does not mean that she is a lady; and there you have *he,* but not necessarily a man. This *he* and *she* are something much higher than creation and what is represented as male or female here on Earth. It is the eternal *he* and the eternal *she* that meet us in these substances, and this division is a real necessity here. However, just as here on Earth the *he* is often unable to live without the *she*, and vice versa, silica can be understood only when it works together with the lime, and the lime can be understood only when it works with the silica. The crust of the Earth consists of fifty percent silica, and thirty percent lime. Imagine what this means. Imagine that wherever we walk, *he* and *she* have provided the ground on which we walk. *He,* because he gradually became satisfied; *she,* because she surrendered herself for the possibility that other substances, powers, forces, beings can work through and with her.[80]

All the mollusks build a shell of calcium around their bodies, but only because they are too sensitive; they have so much *she* that they can't do otherwise than make *him* very strong. You will repeatedly find calcium and silica working together in this way.

Don't think that the mussel or the snail are in any way typical *he* images of nature. Just the opposite. This withdrawal, this "don't touch me" is a picture of silica. This is *she;* this is the virgin on the crystal mountain. But if *she* has to enter life, what does she do? She

---

80 König, *Earth and Man*, pp. 235–236.

takes the hard coat of *him*, lime, and puts it around her. Otherwise the equilibrium would be disturbed. You find even in the plant world that the most tender ones have the hardest bark. Don't think that the oak is as unbending as the Teutonic people would like it to be; not in the least. The oak is an immensely tender being.[81]

Although a tremendous amount of lime is precipitated in our skeleton, the form into which it is precipitated is silica. All those beautiful, ingeniously arranged fibers in our bones are built by silica. Once they have formed, they are filled with calcium and the silica disappears. It recedes and the lime takes hold, becomes satisfied, and the bone is built.[82]

We see the picture of silica with its forces gently coming from the periphery, from the outside, the cosmos. From without, these forces are centrifugal, and the lime movement is from within outward, from the center to outside, greedily demanding, radiating centripetal forces. Both work together in harmony, the silica moving in from outside, and the lime moving in filling the layers with its substance.

One can now observe nature and how different plants live in different environments. When I lived in new Hampshire, the granite state, we lived on top of a granite mountain and in August we would go blueberry picking and bring home buckets and buckets for winter's use. The berries grow wild on this silica ground: silica blueberries. They are not acidic, but more alkaline based. Nature is balancing itself out. Where silica is, *she* then *he* comes in the form of delicious blueberries.

In the Bahamas, however, where I spend quite a bit of time in the family of islands, it is the exact opposite. The islands are made from calcium deposits, and lemons and grapefruits grow there like weeds. All acid fruits find their homes. The *he* ground is home to *she*, acid fruits. On the sandy soils up in Maine one finds a beautiful

---

81   Ibid., p. 239.

82   Ibid., p. 241.

flower with a majestic bean-like flower, a bean plant gesture full of nitrogen. The desert is home to the sweetest dates, and so forth.

One can begin looking at the environment with this picture in mind. It provides a beginning for understanding the plant kingdom as well as the animal kingdom. The forces coming from the periphery, the cosmos, and the forces coming from the center are basic to an understanding of our world, and therefore to the foods we choose to eat.

> Neither calcium nor silica nourishes living organisms. They feed neither the plant world, nor animals, nor human beings. Nevertheless, they are necessary for the whole world.
>
> If they are not nourishment, what are they? It is very difficult to describe what they are, but perhaps you will understand what I mean when I say they are catalysts. They do not change themselves, but they must be present, and in their presence all others, or many other substances, start to order and arrange themselves in the proper way.[83]

One can start by noticing where one lives. Is it granite, silica, or is it calcium and lime deposited ages ago from retiring seas? Or is it clay made of aluminum compounds, or sandy, or the beautiful dark humus earth of the Midwest? Then we can begin analyzing rock formations and the trees that grow near us and by doing so we learn about our place and what we are taking in from our surroundings.

Do people who live on top of granite mountains think more clearly? Is the silica going to help me in my spiritual work? For me, I believe the answer is yes. If I lived on sandy or lime soil, what would that mean? What does it mean to live on ground that is lime, with its incredible drawing-up forces? I have experienced both, and one can see they are completely different from one another, if one learns how to be quiet enough to notice.

---

83 Ibid., p. 234.

Now I am surrounded by high peaks, with granite and alluvial glacial deposits, riverbeds, and clay. Is this helping me in my work? I think so; otherwise I would not be here. People are called to live in different areas that coincide with their inner destiny, but it is helpful to understand how we are affected. If something is not going right, perhaps a change of scenery is necessary for one's wellbeing. That is extremely important for the life of a young family, and their health depends on it. If the husband comes home exhausted and is not doing well, or the wife complains of health issues, perhaps relocation is necessary. Consulting with an anthroposophic doctor is also very helpful.

What is the difference if one lives in an oak savannah or a maple woods, or in pine and birch country? I have lived in all of the above, and they all bring distinct feelings. Now I prefer the tall pine, spruce, cedar forests with birch trees here and there. But I do miss maple trees.

But what does this have to do with food? As we have discussed in some detail, we receive our nourishment from the cosmos. From the periphery it comes into our twelve senses. Here I feed myself on cedar groves, pine trees, birch trees; they become my main nutrients for several months, along with high mountain peaks.

If we look at where we live with these insights we will be very surprised to learn a lot more about ourselves, which is the reason for mentioning all of this. Readers may start thinking a bit about their environment, the minerals they walk upon, the plants they live with and consume, and the animal kingdom that accompanies them on their journey.

Now we will jump to what appears to be a totally different subject, but it is not. Living with such a picture as calcium-silica is extremely important, as you will note from the following passage. If we live fully in our environment, this also has an impact on our future.

It actually makes a great difference whether people pay attention to things in life, whether they take an interest in every detail, or whether they do not pay attention to things....

Everything in which the whole body takes part, when human beings are attentive and observant, passes over into the structure of the head of the next earthly life, and has a definite effect.... The head has a strong tendency to develop a strong relationship to the forces of the Earth. What happens then?...The result is that in such human beings there is a special development of everything that depends on the forces of the Earth. They get large, strong bones, extremely broad shoulder blades, for instance, and the ribs are well developed. Everything bears the stamp of good development....

People whose karma it is in the next earthly life to have strong bones and well developed muscles as the result of attentiveness to life—such people...go through life with courage. Through their attentiveness they have also acquired the natural force that belongs to a courageous life.[84]

From such deep insights, we can see that strong bones are not all about calcium. We earn them through a deep interest in the world, and not by taking calcium pills or drinking milk. The other aspect is this:

Now let us think of cowardly, fainthearted people. They are those who took no interest in anything during the previous earthly life.... However, if we go through our present earthly life with a certain amount of self-knowledge, then we can prepare for the *next* earthly life. If we drift superficially through life, without taking an interest in anything, we can be sure that we will be cowards in the next earthly life. This is because a detached, inattentive character forms few links with its environment and, consequently, the head organization in the next life lacks any relationship with the forces of the Earth. The bones remain undeveloped, the hair grows slowly: very often such a person has bowed legs or knock knees.[85]

---

84 Steiner, *Karmic Relationships*, vol. 6, pp. 122–123.

85 Ibid., vol. 2, p. 124.

AFRICA

Africa is a large continent, undergoing massive changes and painful events through famine, wars, and dry conditions. It seems the continent is dying. It can't seem to rejuvenate itself.

It is the home of millet, a grain rich in iron. The colors that one sees in Africa are totally different from those of other continents. It is made up of earthen colors, deep brown, black, indigo, golden yellow, brilliant orange, which made people's beautiful black and coffee-toned skin appear even richer. It is an earthy continent as opposed to the green temperate zones. The people here live in their limbs, displaying a beautiful strength unmatched in the West. It becomes apparent when we watch the Olympics and see the runners' and other athletes' well developed muscles. We can see the body type of the Chinese, and then we can understand the power that resides in the African body. It seems because of the power of the Sun heating the African continent with force, its people have grown more into their limbs than the rest of us. They are superb athletes as a result, and very much incarnated into their bodies, as opposed to floating up in the heavens like the lithe Chinese.

JAPAN

One cannot talk about food without mentioning sushi bars, brown rice, tofu, Zen Buddhism, macrobiotics, tea ceremony, Japanese gardens, green tea, plum blossoms, algae, juice bars—the list goes on.

The East has taken the West by surprise, bringing welcome change to the northern American diet that we spoke about earlier. It counteracts all the malefic effect of the potatoes, meat, corn, sugar, and milk, and goes to the other end of the spectrum. It brings a revolution in diet that the American continent needs to create a balance. We can now look at the ingredients, once again, and what forces stand behind them.

We spoke about rice, but with brown rice we have the addition of untreated rice whose roughage and fiber will help cleanse the colon, the intestines, of putrefied matter. For someone who is changing their diet, what brown rice gives is essential to cleansing and making the digestive system work at acquiring its own starches in a slow manner. This will strengthen the digestive process rather than weaken it by giving it white rice and refined foods. Tofu brings the protein element into the diet, and later we will address what could be a concern with a strictly no-meat, no-eggs, and no-milk product diet replaced by tofu products, especially for the younger generation and women in particular.

Tofu is made from soybeans, and soybeans come from the bean family. To reiterate: proteins are made of carbon-hydrogen-oxygen, plus nitrogen and sulfur. Carbon-hydrogen-oxygen are the ingredients of carbohydrates. Grain has ten percent protein; legumes have twenty-five percent protein.

We touched lightly on the subject of proteins with our discussions of India and legumes (lentils), stimulants in South America, nitrogen in nightshade foods, and peanuts. Now we can go a bit further into the soya beans that grow on gigantic farms in the Midwest along with corn. One year corn is planted, and then the next, soybeans, and so forth. Enormous amounts of fertilizers are applied to the soil so that the whole continent is being poisoned, and it is a matter of time before the plants become so weak that their nutritional values will be zero, regardless of human manipulation of the seeds. The tons of pesticides applied and food's increasing emptiness are results of the great demand for soybean products, and this demand is the direct result of the revolutionary influence of Japanese food on our diet. Like everything else, one needs to look at the positive as well as the negative and then make a decision about what we eat, which is what this book is about, along with the stories. The stories are not the point, but are just the medium I use to make the more difficult material more digestible, accessible, and reader-friendly. They also help because a picture of a food when it is seen in an original setting will stand out in someone's memory, and then forces and chemical phenomena behind the particular foods will be easier to retain or understand. I am a painter and I love pictures, but don't be fooled. Behind all the stories there is *powerful knowledge.*

Returning to the soya beans, I call this plant the new queen of foods. After living in the Midwest for many years I have seen it planted early every spring, watched it grow and then harvested by huge tractors. I have seen this harvest loaded into long-haul trailer trucks, some of it sometimes spilling onto the country roads for the crows or the local deer population to eat.

This new Queen Soya contains a lot of protein, twenty-five percent, and that is her signature. Proteins represent the prototype, the bearer, of life. *Proteos* is the Greek word for "first." Unlike fats and sugars, it cannot be stored. Sugar is stored in the form of glucose in the liver, and fat—well you know where fats goes, unfortunately for some.

> Protein...is constantly subjected to renewal in the organism.... Protein therefore cannot be stored or conserved as can fats and carbohydrates. It constantly changes, coming and going;...protein is always on the point either of being taken into activity of the etheric body or of falling away from it. This leads to the constant building up and breaking down of protein in the organism, to the need to be renewed daily through nutrition, as well as excreted every day....
>
> Protein in the ganglia of the brain is renewed on average every nine hours. The so called half-life enzymes (made of proteins) are likewise only a few hours. In the liver, it takes about ten days for its protein to be renewed, whereas for the muscles it takes 150 days.... Thus, the most varying rhythms of building up and breaking down protein hold sway in the organism. We come to the body of formative forces (ether/plant body) expressed in the protein activity.[86]

---

86 Schmidt, *Essentials of Nutrition*, p. 52.

Gerhard Schmidt then goes on to point out the separation of proteins into "globular proteins" contained in egg cell formation, reproduction, blood and enzymes, and the "scleroprotein," which make up the collagen in tendons, cartilage, or connective tissues.

We have a polarity within proteins. We know that earlier forms of life such as oysters and lobsters have a strong reproductive life and protein activity, the embryo being at the center of this activity, but next to this reproductive activity are the nerve-sense cells.

> Wherever I think or feel, I do so with the same forces that exercise formative activity in the lower animals or in the plant world....
>
> Protein thus comes into the "upper human" under the influence of forces that push back this plasticity. Proteins are transformed into the soul's ability to think and feel. The protein itself is transformed in its character and structure. It becomes scleroprotein, appropriate to the building up of form and frame.... The greatest imaginable care must be taken, that neither too little nor too much protein is taken into the body.[87]

As the bearer of life, protein is indispensable. Nonetheless, it must not hinder the other pole of the human being, that of consciousness. One has to be reminded that protein is made up of the same thing as carbohydrates. But add nitrogen. That is oxygen, hydrogen, and carbon plus nitrogen.

Now we see that protein is essential to life, to the reproduction of life, and to the human being's life of thought. Proteins, the nitrogen force which we discussed earlier in the poisonous plants, allow for a life of sensitivity, allow us to be thinking human beings. Protein has both abilities, these two incredible polarities: *life and death*—life in the reproduction mode and death in the forming of consciousness. The activity of the oysters, shrimp, and lower creatures, which is full of life as we see in the incredible rate at which they reproduce themselves, is transformed into *our* ability to feel

---

87 Ibid., pp. 51–53.

and think, which is a *death process*. This picture needs to be lived with and meditated upon in order to truly understand proteins.

Now we can go further. We mentioned at the beginning that in our digestive system we must break down foods, destroy them entirely, create chaos, and then humanize the substance again with our own "I"-forces. When we cannot digest something, that is when we poison ourselves, because we do not have enough strength to destroy the ingested substances. The substances come to a zero point, and then our humanness comes into the picture and humanizes the substances. One with a strong, higher "I" will not have digestive problems. Steiner mentioned in a joking way at some lectures, especially to the female audience, the fact that if one learned how to think, or apply their thinking ability, they would not be fat in their next incarnation. He meant that a stronger "I," one who can think rather than wallow in feelings, will have stronger forces to digest fat and use it. The fat evaporates into *thinking*. Now back to proteins and soybeans and their overconsumption.

> Substances such as hemoglutin,[88] which can be found in soybeans, led Pythagoras to the important saying, "Keep away from beans!" They are alien to the actual nature of plants. They have taken an animal-like quality, and we are not able to deal with them; they become a hindering force in us when we eat them. Let us remember that the "artificial meat" developed in the West is made of soya precisely because it is similar to animal flesh. Here, the West has taken something from the East, something that also belongs to the character of the Western materialistic striving for health. Even a so-called vegetarian is thus able to have artificial meat from soybeans, prepared with chicken breast flavor![89]

> Humanity today does not need rules, knowledge and insight; not fixed traditions, but the development of new capacities; not an

---

88 Unfermented soy is high in hemoglutin, which causes clumping of red blood cells and may increase risk of stroke.

89 Schmidt, *Essentials of Nutrition*, p. 306.

escapist "key to the Kingdom of Heaven," but to carry the spiritual into the earthly realm.[90]

The other plant used in this diet is algae. It is used to wrap rice for sushi and is found in many other dishes as well. Algae, as we know, are very ancient plants—remnants of former times. They are very rich in iodine and various other nutrients; however, as ancient plants they are not suitable for our present consciousness. If we study the plant world and its evolution, plants evolve as we do. The plants that are more our friends—those that have evolved with us and are not remnants of previous cycles—are plants such as the crucifers (broccoli etc.), labiates (aromatic herbs), *Umbelliferae* (celery, carrot, parsley family), and grains. We also have mushrooms, which are ancient, parasitic plants and yeasts. They are primitive and not as developed as the later plants that have a sound root system and developed foliage. Those primitive plants affect the brain, because it is the most ancient part of our body. Certainly, we might want to use the primitive plants for certain ailments, but not in our regular diet. Steiner gives us some indication about karma:

> In the case of illnesses, therefore, when we see how far back the influential events lie, karma can indicate to us that an affection, say, of the legs comes from incarnations in the relatively near past, whereas a symptom of illness in the head comes from incarnations in the relatively far distant past....
>
> The results of this are extremely important for therapy. Where should we look for a remedy for illness affecting the head or illness affecting the legs? The remedy for illness affecting the head will be found in what existed far back in the evolutionary process of nature, in what recalls very early natural processes—for instance, mushrooms, which in their present imperfect form recapitulate an earlier plant formation; in algae and lichens; or, in the case of the fully developed plant, in the root, since that is the part that has remained at the earliest stage. Illness in the lower body and more

---

90 Ibid., p. 299.

toward its periphery will have to be healed with what appeared at a later stage in the evolution of nature—blossoms, flowering plants, or later formations in the mineral kingdom.[91]

We need the sunnier plants—sunflower seeds, for example, or apples, carrots, spinach, kale, yams, radishes, beets, corn, and the other plants growing in our temperate zones. Here is more about the primal plants:

> Finally, we may consider the frequent recommendation for algae to be used as human nutrition.... Algae were used in prehistoric times as food, both in the Far East and in the far West among the Aztecs. Even today, algae products play a significant role in the diet of the average Japanese person. These facts have led to the establishment of research projects dealing with the breeding of various species of algae for human consumption. One is attracted to the idea of finding substances that, in addition to their high protein content, are also rich in vitamins and minerals. But one important fact is not considered; we are dealing with a very old plant formation. It originated in the distant past of the Earth. At that time, human beings were still far from their later and present organization. The forces of these plants correspond in no way to the level of development humanity has attained since then. Although algae from ancient times are still used as food today, one should see— through modern consciousness—that an algae-based diet is no longer appropriate. Algae correspond to a level of development that leads to decadence today, not toward progress. This statement is meant in the light of something we have often emphasized—human nutrition works not only on our corporeal nature, but also on our consciousness. It is exactly from this point of view that we must understand why the consumption of algae should not be revived. The protein appropriate to our culture comes more from the green plants rooted in the earth. This leads us primarily to grain proteins.[92]

---

91   Steiner, *Karmic Relationships,* vol. 7, p. 122.
92   Schmidt, *Essentials of Nutrition,* p. 80.

When we find the fossilized creatures that lived long ago, we realize that they could have been like our modern animals and plants, and in particular not like our present plants. All the primeval plants must have been much more like our sponges, mushrooms, and algae. There is a difference between our mushrooms and other plants today, which take in the carbon and form their body from it. When they sink into the ground, their body remains as coal....

Today's plants, including the plants that now provide us with coal, are built up of carbon. Much earlier plants, however, were formed not from carbon but from nitrogen. That was possible because, just as carbon dioxide is exhaled today by animal and human, in ancient times a combination of carbon and nitrogen was exhaled. That is prussic acid, the terribly poisonous hydrocyanic acid fatal to all life today. This poisonous hydrocyanic acid was once exhaled, and nothing that exists today could then have arisen. Early mushroom-like plants took in nitrogen and formed their body from it. The creatures..., the birdlike beings and the heavy, coarse animal-beings, breathed out this poisonous acid, and the plants around them took the nitrogen to form their plant-body. Here, too, we can see that substances still existing today were used in quite a different way in ancient times.[93]

The Japanese people being one of the oldest people on our Earth would include in their diet primitive plants, and such is the case. We Westerners need other diets that are more appropriate for where we stand now. Algae and mushrooms are examples, as they are remnant of former times.

Today we must increasingly develop a consciousness of what we are connecting ourselves to when we eat. Whether they come from the Earth of from the cosmos, we must understand the forces that stimulate us to detoxify, to overcoming illness—in a word, to becoming healthy. We need insight into how our food should be prepared, how much of it should we eat, and how it should be combined.[94]

---

93 Steiner, *From Sunspots to Strawberries...*, pp. 43–44.
94 Schmidt, *Essentials of Nutrition*, p. 308.

THE MIDDLE EAST

Now I would like to discuss Mount Sinai, the Dead Sea, salt, and minerals once again. I find these fascinating, especially the phrase, "You are the salt of the earth."

I could never really understand this sentence. Why are human beings called "the salt of the earth"? Why not sugar, or diamonds, or gold? I have lived with that question for many years, and now that I have taken this food and nutrition journey, the old saying has new meaning. The other is "The man was made from a lump of *clay*": adamah–earth–clay, the first human. All these minerals remind me of Mt. Sinai for some reason. I guess it is the biblical reference, the Dead Sea, and all the rocks. It reminds me of the desert, Moses, and Israel. What it has to do with nutrition came to me later. It has to do with *salt* and, of course, *thinking.*

I had a chance to bathe in the Dead Sea several times during my stay, and believe me it is salty and one cannot drown, which is lucky for people who can't swim. I was warned not to plunge into the water, which I love to do, and I am glad I did not. I would have been blinded by the salt in my eyes. But I enjoyed the heavy waters and did like everyone else. I put layers of clay mud on myself and baked in the sunlight. I then rinsed myself, and did it again. It is excellent for the skin, and people say it rejuvenates it, so I rejuvenated myself thoroughly along with many Israelis coming from Tel Aviv or Jerusalem or the United States, and elsewhere. The Bronx was heavily represented, as was Long Island, Manhattan, New York City, Madrid, Paris, Rome, and Munich, all chatting in every language imaginable. Palestinians who were lucky enough to come out of their barbed wire enclave were swimming in their birkini, meaning "burka kini." I enjoyed it all, and hoped that my 62-year-old skin did too. People were selling creams for everything you could think of. Being French, I have a love for beauty creams. Ask my close friends. There were creams with clay, salt, and perfumes—food for the skin.

I bought nothing, because I had it for free on the beach, but I bought some creams in Cairo where it was cheaper.

Here we see that clay goes with salt, and Moses was just up the road through the desert, past the frontier, and into Egypt. We have mentioned silica and limestone in the story of *he and she*, and phosphorus when we talked about rice. But now, since we are encountering the salty sea and this marvelous, healing substance clay-*adamah*-earth, let us look more closely at this clay.

Silica is an acid, and limestone is a base. When base and acid unite they form salt. With this substance clay, which is made out of aluminum, it can unite either with an acid or a base. It is able to move between these substances, acid and base (he and she), and create a balance. We can see this activity of aluminum, or clay, in the planet Earth.

Silica is responsible for color, scent (she), and finely articulated form, whereas lime (he) sees to the material filling-out of vegetation from below. Aluminum keeps these earthly and heavenly forces in living balance. That is why we called *luxuriance of foliage*—the green middle zone of the plant kingdom—a sure indication of a clay-rich soil.

Clay is plastic and responsive to formative forces working on it from outside. Just as a musical instrument responds to a musician, so plastic clay is the instrument for the music of forms composed by a sculptor.

It is the aluminum process that makes Earth receptive to the cosmic shaping forces of the silica process (she), which the great artist, Nature, draws from the cosmic periphery. Silica's affinity to water appears again here in relationship to clay, for it is only when clay is properly moist that it is sufficiently plastic to be receptive to the shaping activity of silica....

We might say...that human beings are built from head to toe from the balance of heavenly and earthly forces that clay affords. But this "clay" undergoes a step-by-step upward purifying as human beings refine it in their various organs, reaching a peak in the eye's transparency; here dark earthly matter has been lifted to a level where it becomes permeable by the light of the spirit.[95]

We must not forget that most precious stones are made of aluminum oxide and compounds of aluminum; rubies and sapphires are pure aluminum oxide. In these beautiful stones, the perfect balance is achieved thanks to aluminum, between the silica and the lime.

Clay is made of aluminum. Aluminum is a latecomer in the metals kingdom. It is extremely difficult to extract from its compounds, unlike silver and copper compounds. It is only because of our technological advances that we have aluminum. The metal is now used everywhere, even in cooking, but one should stay away from using aluminum cooking pots; it is better to use steel.

> In nature, aluminum occurs primarily as clay, aluminum oxide, combined in manifold ways with other substances. Thus it has an important share of the formation of rock and of fertile soil. Without aluminum there would be no fertile earth. In the oldest igneous rocks it occurs as feldspar....
>
> Since about sixty percent of the Earth's rock mass is feldspar, it is clear that aluminum is not only the most widely distributed but also, quantitatively, the most abundant metal....
>
> [Clay] conveys to the soil the properties of plasticity and water absorption; the ability to unite with the living substance that is water, and to surrender to the plastic formative forces. Such is aluminum's role as a mediator. It is the instrument of a "mineral/plant" nature.... With its help the forces of the inner Earth are carried upward into the plant world that unfolds upon the surface.[96]

Clay performs the action of uniting both the *he and she*. It unites the opposites.

---

95   Hauschka, *Nature of Substance*, p. 134.
96   Pelikan, *The Secrets of Metals*, pp. 190–192.

Aluminum unites the life-bearing water with the earthly element that is to be plastically formed. It is a bond between the siliceous and the calcareous in the mineral world.... [It] is in a certain way...the rhythmical metal of the mineral world.[97]

It is no wonder clay is associated with humanity. As humans, we unite the Earth with the heavens as in aluminum, the new metal that does not like to be a metal but likes to unite with all the elements, the he and the she. It is a worthy example for us to follow. It is active within our blood and circulation. Our blood contains minute quantities of *all the metals*; aluminum is only one of them.

I always wear precious stones, not as a way of showing wealth, but because I have always learned much from them. I have been wearing a beautiful ruby for many years now. The ruby is related to the force of intuition. It is made of aluminum oxide as is the sapphire, which is related to our destiny, our "feet." We see that clay can become beautiful precious stones, emeralds included, like the carbon becomes a diamond. Aluminum becomes sapphires, rubies, and emeralds. They unite Earth and Heaven, and their imperfections become the bright red, blue, or green from specks of minerals in the stones. It is said that wearing a moonstone will bring on childbirth and will help in bringing a child into this world.

At the beginning of a nation, Moses led by rules in order to control the wild passionate forces that still dominated the souls and bodies of human beings, to tame animalistic impulses, and to make bodies that would be fit to house the spirit of a savior, Christ. To this day, orthodox Jews follow rules to conduct their life, including dietary rules such as *Kashrut*. These rules are unquestioned. They say, "God wanted it!"

One of the main rules is that meat and dairy may not be eaten together. That rule seems very fair: not eating the animal that provided one with the milk products. It shows respect and a certain

---

97 Ibid., p. 92.

restraint. If followed by more people, that rule would save a lot of food, and this could feed others who are not so fortunate.

The other rule, making sure the meat has no blood, is also a good rule to follow. It means the body does not ingest the blood, the animalistic bloody flesh. This rule makes it easier to digest and spiritually keeps the body clear of animalistic impulses.

The aspect of using different kitchen utensils for cooking meat and vegetarian or milk dishes acknowledges the fact that there are residues—spiritual aspects to eating meat—that should not be mixed with vegetables and milk. It stains the one with the other, again trying to keep the body pure of the animalistic aspects of meat. The rules make it easier to keep a clean body, but do they help keep the soul clean?

In our day and age people must work on their inner selves in order to purify themselves through meditative work. Then the rules become unnecessary. I do not feel like eating the meat of the cow and then drinking her milk; it seems overdoing it. But I came to that conclusion on my own. Why do I need protein from the milk when I already have the protein from the meat?

By counting on dietary laws in order to keep the body pure, one accepts the fact that one is weak and unable to do anything about purity. In the 21st century it is atavistic, and furthermore, it makes human beings think they are not responsible for themselves. People need rules when they are not strong enough to obey their inner conscience. We are supposed to go beyond the rules, keeping our boundaries within ourselves so we need not be told what to do. Otherwise we remain at a childish stage of evolution.

One of my favorite recipes that comes from the Ukraine is for borsht, which my children also love. Another is for dumplings. I had a wonderful time eating in Jerusalem among the vendors in the bazaar, or in the wealthy Jewish quarter, or the Christian orthodox section. The foods were very similar to each other.

I stayed in the monastery of St. Catherine next to Mt. Sinai, and a friend and I were fortunate to climb the famous mountain in the morning with no one else around. In our solitude, my mind could wander within this biblical setting. The rocks in this ancient telluric center feel volcanic and evoke a fiery atmosphere. It seems dry and lifeless, unfriendly and so earthly it is not earthly. It was stormy even though the Sun was shining. It is no wonder, I thought, that Moses chose this area. It is said that geology and rocks dominate the destiny of the Hebrews. This is the place then, on top of the mountains, the birth of the Hebrew nation, the beginning of the emancipation from the gods. I lay on the rocks and impregnated myself with the overwhelming rocky, toothy peaks, imagining the sight of Moses and his people. These were desert tribal people, shepherds, former believers in many gods, practicing all sorts of decadent worship rituals. At this place he was to bring them in line in a forceful manner with rules and regulations that aimed to tame those wild animalistic forces. Perhaps the beginning of hatred toward and subjugation of women began here under the dominance of this patriarchal system. It reigned in the wild, stormy, passionate sexual forces with rules, and women were made into slaves. There was fear of women and their sexual powers. This began the Moslem, Christian, and Jewish subjugation of women by covering them up and keeping them hidden from view.[98] Now I will return to the subject of food.

❧

I was driving through Israel with a friend and it was late at night, not far from the Dead Sea and Jordan. We were tired so we turned off on some desert road. It was dark so we could not see anything except that it was some kind of farm. We stopped and an older, polite man came out. We chatted and said we needed a place to stay. They were farmers, industrial farmers. As we waited for the polite

---

98 This is the subject of my next book, *Beyond the Blood*.

man, who had been in the United States, to make phone calls, we noticed that small tractors were returning to the farm with people on them who had their faces covered with handkerchiefs. I was puzzled because it was late to be working. They showed their faces and I could see they were men and women from the Far East. I couldn't understand it; they looked Vietnamese or at least from that part of the world. We finally got a place down the road, which was a tent-like family youth hostel for people from Tel Aviv who wanted a bit of relaxation. It was constructed for those who have dozens of children. The kids were able to run around and give their parents some peace.

They gave us a little room next door to some Russians kids who were watching a movie in Russian—all night. So we got no sleep. The Russians were also working there. In the morning, I had a talk with the owner, a handsome fit Israeli with a beautiful, tanned wife, who took a vacation every year to South America. I saw that the huge vegetable and herb farms under plastic were staffed by imported foreign laborers. These farms were doing enormous trade with European countries, especially with peppers, tomatoes, cucumbers, and a new market for herbs. All were shipped across the ocean. They said that their main competitors were the Spaniards. At the same time the Palestinians, who had wonderful food stands by the side of the road with organically grown produce, were prevented from selling their products in the local cities.

I asked about water and he laughed, saying there was plenty of water. We were in the middle of the desert, the Dead Sea, but they had enormous pumps in wells going very deep, taking water from the underground deposit. This was just a few miles across the desert from Jordan, a place that also needs the water. These agricultural practices were certainly not organic, and seemed run by slave labor, people who have no say in anything, and the crops were sold to unknowing markets in Europe.

This is a realm in which the homemaker can make choices. One must know where food comes from and how it is grown. Who works there? In South and Central America we have the beginnings of fair trade, but in the Middle East it is nonexistent, and companies go to great lengths to cover up how and where the food is grown.

When shopping for food I always ask where it comes from. I buy locally at all times and try to get the produce from the gardeners in my region if I am not living on the farm. The best alternative is to establish a community farm. This is not easy, but now we do not have a choice if we want our children to grow healthy. The corporate foods are not to be trusted. The local farm movement is a healthy one and should be supported. Much work needs to be done, but that is how we change.

PART 3: CONCLUSION: FUTURE LANDS

As the reader may have noticed, I love traveling and observing people and their customs, and I will continue my travels to places I have not yet been. I often do an exercise—taking the whole Earth into my consciousness and focusing on a specific country I have visited, reliving in my mind what that particular place imprinted into my soul. I then have a great love for the Earth as a being rather than a place with imaginary lines of demarcation and countries that should exist in the first place. This way I keep in touch with a wholeness that belongs to our Earth, and I go beyond race, nationalistic feelings, and language. These things separate humankind. Instead of fragmentation, I encounter wholeness. This food journey has been an exercise in reliving these rich environments with their varied religions, cultures, foods, geography, and people and it has brought me new inspiration and warmth. But behind all its various elements, people everywhere are all human beings with similar feelings: love for their family, language, geography, culture, and religion that they are free to practice without coercion.

But there are areas where intransigent demands have created hatred instead of cooperation and segregation instead of sharing. These areas will become extinct in the future, as people will abandon them for places where an atmosphere of freedom and cooperation exist. If one spreads hate, on gets it back; such is the law of karma. Hate in one lifetime becomes suffering and stupidity in the next incarnation. Steiner mentions that if you hate a particular race or people you *will incarnate* into that race, just to learn not to hate. We have more than one life.

If we look at all the areas where hate is rampant, then we see that many of these human beings will be reborn with enormous suffering and stupidity. By the same token, where there is enormous suffering, it is a sign that there was hate in previous lives. It is a vicious cycle, which the younger generation is trying to break. The attraction to the lifestyle of places like the United States, Canada, Western Europe, and Australia is because these places share space with people from multiple racial, linguistic, and religious backgrounds. Diverse people meet and work together in hospitals, universities, industries, and the arts, and work in cooperation with each other. They share and learn about one another's foods, music, and religious practices and thereby become a brotherhood and sisterhood of humankind rather than a system of patriarchy or religious affiliation. Brothers and sisters are different from fathers and mothers.

When I travel I usually do not socialize with the intelligentsia or upper class. I make it a rule. I meet the locals, the people who work, those who live close to the land, or those who use their own hands to make a living. They are the ones I meet in the far-off corners of the Earth. They invite me into their homes and they share a meal, bread, whatever they have, and I share some of my own dates, nuts, and cheese. We share something that is human. There is no profit or status in these meetings, no reciprocity, but genuine sharing, a concept our Western world has forgotten. The West is about money, and brotherhood or sisterhood are difficult when money is involved. The people I meet are the forgotten ones; no one cares if they have enough food. They are content with just a little food while the politicians are too busy thinking of themselves and lining their pockets. When the going gets rough for them they send out the tanks.

I have seen enormous estates everywhere; thousands of acres in the United States are owned by thieves. Everywhere locals work for nothing and owners sit in some parliament somewhere, whether it is in Spain, France, Italy, Morocco, Tunisia, Israel, or Egypt. There are enormous farms and industries of all kinds: citrus fruit farms, pig farms, cattle ranches, olive plantations owned by Saudi princes, mines, and industrial complexes, and one cannot fathom their wealth. Next door, people are living on nothing but are happy with a couple of camels or a few pigs, or a dozen or so olive and fruits trees in the middle of the desert, using ingenious techniques.

But in some little pockets of the Earth, brotherhood and sisterhood can be found. When you sit on a dirt floor in a mud home with a cup of tea, or someone in the middle of nowhere in Spain or France invites you for a coffee because you are exhausted and have a long way to go, that is a beginning. This means far more than a meal in a restaurant with a person who has a fat bank account to discuss "busy-ness," meaning "you help me, I help you."

When we partake of a meal, especially if that meal is not the food we are accustomed to, we share a little bit of someone else's psyche, someone else's geography and culture. We make the effort to go beyond ourselves and reach into the other with no agenda, certainly not a monetary or deal-making agenda. That is a beginning of brother- and sisterhood. This book was an attempt to do that.

These words by Georg Kühlewind, a Hungarian scientist, master of meditation, survivor of the holocaust, teacher of many (including me) across borders and religious denominations, speak the truth about our world. (*Ego*, here, refers to our lower, selfish self.)

The "I" gives, the ego takes. The destructiveness of the ego is immediately evident in social terms: *everyone* wants to take, to have, and the result is discord and warfare. Today we are experiencing the collapse of a social system based on egoism both in the East and in the West. Long ago the fanatic belief of economic liberalism (that if the individual strives for maximum economic prosperity the result will be maximum prosperity for all) has been shown to be wishful thinking, an ideology meant to somehow socially justify gross egoism. The answer to liberalism was hardly better. Marx never discovered that individual egoism cannot be overcome through class egoism. Class egoism, national egoism, or the egoism of the individual: they all lead to a general defeat in a war of all against all. No social contract helps here. An agreement as to the socially necessary limits on egoism is as ineffective as an agreement on *Realpolitik* as a basis for marriage. Ambition against ambition, greed against greed, will-to-power against will-to-power—how can this lead anywhere but to continual conflict?

Egoism is not only socially destructive; it is also a disease for the individual. Humankind has the use of free word energies. It would be healthy for people to use these *as* word energies—that is, a healthy life would be a creative life. Not everyone has to be a poet, sculptor, or scientist: everyone is creative who radiates peace and the warmth of love and evokes these in others. Such people, mostly quite unknown women and men—not artists, not "personalities"—are the real helpers of humankind....

Egoism means that one's attention is divided: a large portion is directed toward oneself, toward the effect and results of one's activity, not toward the activity itself, or the matter at hand.... When people are self-concerned, as in egotism, they cannot realize a healthy, creative existence. Creation is a pleasure—the greatest of all pleasures.[1]

We have spoken about many different aspects of food, earthly and cosmic food, and how it affects us. We, as human beings, will evolve and continue evolving. As we battle our own selfishness for thousands of years to come, what will we be like in the future? As we go beyond egoism, crass selfishness, and evolve to being selfless, brotherly, and caring, here are some insights given by Rudolf Steiner about the future, the very far-off future. But that future lies within our own life now; we are creating our future, *now*, and what we *do* now is the future:

All that goes on in the soul changes the organism. Imagine people who are able to create their own likenesses through the spoken word, whose hearts have become a voluntary muscle, who will have altered yet other organs. Then you have a conception of the future of the human race in future planetary incarnations of Earth.

---

1 Kühlewind, *From Normal to Healthy*, pp. 72–73.

Humanity will progress on our Earth as far as it is possible under the influence of the mineral kingdom. This mineral kingdom, in spite of having arisen the last, will be the first to disappear again in its present form. Human beings will then no longer build up their bodies from mineral substances as today. The coming human body will only incorporate into itself substances of a plant nature. All that works in human beings today as mineral will disappear. Here is a seemingly grotesque example: today we spit out our ordinary saliva. It is a mineral product, for the physical body is an interaction of mineral processes. When human beings have ended their mineral evolution they will no longer have mineral spittle; it will be of a plant nature—people will, so to speak, spit flowers. Glands will no longer secrete what is mineral, but only a vegetable substance. The mineral kingdom will be brought to an end by the evolutionary return of humanity to vegetable, plant existence.

Thus human beings will pass on to Jupiter, by expelling all that is mineral and progressing to the creativeness of the plant. Later still they will pass over to animal-creativeness—animals will be different from those of today—when their hearts will have progressed so far that they can appear as creators. Then human beings will create in the animal world as today they create in the mineral kingdom; this is when the Venus incarnation will arise. When human beings can create their kind by virtue of uttering their own likeness, then will the meaning of evolution be complete, then will the words be fulfilled: "Let us make humanity in our image, after our likeness."

Only by observing this aspect—that the body will be moulded by the soul—will human beings really transform the human race.... What humanity thinks today, that will it be in the future. A humanity that thinks materialistically will produce frightful beings in the future, and a humanity that thinks spiritual thoughts will work in such a way upon the future organism, transforming it, that beautiful human bodies will proceed from it.

What the materialistic mode of thought brings about has not yet been completed. We have two streams today, a great materialistic one which fills the Earth, and a small spiritual one which is restricted to a few human beings. Distinguish between soul-evolution and race-evolution. Do not think that if races pass over to a grotesque form, the soul, too, will do the same. All materialistic thinking souls work on the production of evil race-formations, and what is done of a spiritual nature causes the bringing forth of a good race. Just as humanity has brought forth creations that have retrogressed as animals, plants, and minerals, so will a portion split off and represent the evil part of humanity.... Just as older conditions that have degenerated to the ape species seem grotesque to us today, so will materialistic races remain at the standpoint of evil, peopling the Earth as evil races. It will lie entirely with the human being as to whether a soul wants to remain in the bad race or wants to ascend by spiritual culture to a good race.[2]

This morning on the news a scientist was protesting that science is going too fast and ethical concerns are not keeping up, and the other scientist was all for going full steam ahead. He was referring to the study of genes, or the mapping of DNA, so that we can see what is wrong in our blood and try to fix it through genetic manipulation. The scientist who was all for this type of medical intervention was saying that we need teams of nurses, scientists, and doctors in order to implement the changes that a person wants—change this or that, in order to be ready for the future.

Knowledge such as is included in this book is never considered in such discussions of modern medicine, only what is materialistic. We can see now the result of these manipulations. Rather than acknowledging a spiritual world, which this type of medicine totally ignores, we transform and fool around with the physical body. What kind of human being will evolve out of this nonsense?

Mentioning the future of our human race is not so far-fetched when we consider these kinds of comments on national radio. Money will be diverted to such endeavors with grave consequences. Unless the spiritual is accepted as fact, as it has been in this book, we will

---

2   Steiner, *Rosicrucian Wisdom*, pp. 149–150.

face "Frankenstein medicine," and all sorts of fad diets to promote one thing or another: men and women taking massive vitamins to achieve youthfulness. Unless we try to inform ourselves about real nutrition, as was attempted here, we won't make any progress in achieving real health.

> As a consequence of our mechanistic view of nature, our entire intellectual life has become mechanized and no longer rises to a level that permits thinking about the suprasensory human being. Simultaneously, human souls are becoming "vegetized"—made plant-like and sleepy. Mechanized spirit and "vegetized" soul set the tone of modern cultural life. And when human souls are not warmed by spirit, and human spirits are not illumined by suprasensory cognition, human bodies develop the animalistic qualities now evident in antisocial drives....
>
> Souls pervaded only by this spirit are asleep, like plants, unlike souls warmed through by the true, pulsing will to perceive and value the suprasensory aspect of human nature. These souls learn to behold the divine archetype in every human being and to feel socially responsible toward all. They learn that all human beings on Earth are equal with regard to their innermost soul. On the route leading to the right, *equality* is cultivated by souls warmed through by spirit. When spirit arouses souls from their vegetative state, bodies are ennobled and imbued with an awareness of the suprasensory. These bodies do not become animalistic, but develop real love in the broadest sense. When this happens, individuals recognize themselves as suprasensory beings, who enter earthly bodies in order to learn to love spirit. They also know that earthly bodies need brotherly-sisterly love, because individuals cannot be fully human so long as humanity is without this brotherly-sisterly love.[3]

Goethe, the famous scientist and poet, on his deathbed asked for a humble bowl full of garden soil to be placed at his bedside, so that

---

3   Steiner, *Freedom of Thought and Societal Forces*, pp. 40–41.

he could contemplate the soil, clay, *adamah,* earth. He knew that substances, earth, were the *end of the paths of gods.*

During his life he had done his utmost to remind us of this sacred Earth, how alive it is. He fought all his life against the dead-element, the materialistic approach of scientific thoughts, and he wanted to bring life into our thinking. He knew that his body was returning to the sacred Earth, as his towering spirit was getting ready to return home. How befitting for such a gigantic spirit to contemplate a simple bowl of garden soil.

Earth, like heaven, is shaped by the musical ordering power of the cosmic WORD, which reaches into matter itself and gives it patterns of coherence. Earth is the materialized cosmic word, "the end of God's path."[4]

May our Earth become the home of many more spirits like Goethe. It is our duty to welcome them into the world, and our Earth needs enlightened parents to bring such spirits into the world if they are ready.

⦿

---

4   Hauschka, *Nature of Substance,* p. 232.

BIBLIOGRAPHY

Anonymous. *The Cloud of Unknowing.* San Francisco: HarperOne, 2004.

Hauschka, Rudolf. The *Nature of Substance: Spirit and Matter.* London: Rudolf Steiner Press, 2002.

———. *Nutrition: A Holistic Approach.* London: Rudolf Steiner Press, 2002.

König, Karl. *Earth and Man.* Wyoming, RI: Bio-Dynamic Literature, 1982.

Kühlewind, Georg. *From Normal to Healthy: Paths to the Liberation of Consciousness.* Great Barrington, MA: Lindisfarne Books, 1988.

———. *The Gentle Will: Meditative Guidelines for Creative Consciousness.* Great Barrington, MA: Lindisfarne Books, 2011.

Nasr, Seyyed Hossein. *Islam: Religion, History, and Civilization.* San Francisco: Harper San Francisco, 2003.

Pelikan, Wilhelm. *The Secrets of Metals.* Great Barrington, MA: Lindisfarne Books, 1973.

Schmidt, Gerhard. *The Dynamics of Nutrition.* Wyoming, RI: Bio-Dynamic Literature, 1980.

———. *The Essentials of Nutrition.* Wyoming, RI: Bio-Dynamic Literature, 1987.

Steiner, Rudolf. *Becoming the Archangel Michael's Companions: Rudolf Steiner's Challenge to the Younger Generation.* Great Barrington, MA: SteinerBooks, 2006.

———. *Bees.* Great Barrington, MA: Anthroposophic Press, 1998.

———. *Esoteric Christianity and the Mission of Christian Rosenkreutz.* London: Rudolf Steiner Press, 2000.

———. *Esoteric Lessons, 1904–1909: From the Esoteric School.* Great Barrington, MA: SteinerBooks, 2007.

———. *Freedom of Thought and Societal Forces: Implementing the Demands of Modern Society.* Great Barrington, MA: SteinerBooks, 2008.

———. *From Comets to Cocaine…: Answers to Questions.* London: Rudolf Steiner Press, 2002.

———. *From Crystals to Crocodiles…: Answers to Questions.* London: Rudolf Steiner Press, 2004.

———. *From Mammoths to Mediums…: Answers to Questions.* London: Rudolf Steiner Press, 2000.

———. *From Sunspots to Strawberries…: Answers to Questions.* London: Rudolf Steiner Press, 2002.

———. *Harmony of the Creative Word: The Human Being and the Elemental, Animal, Plant and Mineral Kingdoms.* London: Rudolf Steiner Press, 2007.

———. *Karmic Relationships: Esoteric Studies* (8 vols.). Forrest Row: Rudolf Steiner Press, 1997–2012.

———. *Macrocosm and Microcosm.* London: Rudolf Steiner Press, 1968.

———. *Manifestations of Karma.* London: Rudolf Steiner Press, 1995.

———. *An Outline of Esoteric Science.* Hudson, NY: Anthroposophic Press, 1997.

———. *Rosicrucian Wisdom: An Introduction.* London: Rudolf Steiner Press, 2008.

———. *Start Now! A Book of Soul and Spiritual Exercises.* Great Barrington, MA: SteinerBooks, 2004.

———. *Supersensible Knowledge.* Great Barrington, MA: SteinerBooks, 1987.

———. *Transforming the Soul* (2 vols.). London: Rudolf Steiner Press, 2005–2006.

Valandro, Marie-Laure. *Camino Walk: Where Inner and Outer Paths Meet.* Great Barrington, MA: Lindisfarne Books, 2007.

———. *Deliverance of the Spellbound God: An Experiential Journey into Eastern and Western Meditation Practices.* Great Barrington, MA: Lindisfarne Books, 2011.

———. *Letters from Florence: Observations on the Inner Art of Travel.* Great Barrington, MA: Lindisfarne Books, 2010.

———. *Touched: A Painter's Insights into the Work of Liane Collot d'Herbois.* Great Barrington, MA: Lindisfarne Books, 2012.